How to Perform a Systemat
Literature Review

Edward Purssell • Niall McCrae

How to Perform a Systematic Literature Review

A Guide for Healthcare Researchers, Practitioners and Students

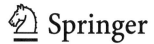 Springer

Edward Purssell 🆔
School of Health Sciences
City, University of London
London
UK

Niall McCrae 🆔
Florence Nightingale Faculty of Nursing
Midwifery & Palliative Care
King's College London
London
UK

ISBN 978-3-030-49671-5   ISBN 978-3-030-49672-2   (eBook)
https://doi.org/10.1007/978-3-030-49672-2

This Springer imprint is published by the registered company Springer Nature Switzerland AG
The registered company address is: Gewerbestrasse 11, 6330 Cham, Switzerland

Contents

Introduction

1

The field of healthcare has undergone, and will continue to undergo, rapid change. Recent events have shown the importance of sharing and understanding data and the need to respond quickly to events. In a hyperconnected world in which a virus can spread throughout the continents in weeks, we no longer need to wait months for print journals to deliver important research findings. Fortunately, we have, in the form of the internet, a tool that enables knowledge to travel around the world at an even faster pace than even the most contagious virus. Quicker and wider access to information, alongside greater transparency in research conduct, should lead to a golden age of evidence-based practice.

However, this information must be managed. The internet is a double-edged sword, as false or dubious claims spread quickly and threaten to undermine the good work of clinicians and researchers, misleading the public and possibly practitioners too. Furthermore, when making decisions that can quite literally be a matter of life or death, it is important that those making these decisions do so using the best available knowledge and also that as knowledge changes so does policy. Acting on partial or poorly understood information can have devastating effects on communities and individuals. When considering a problem, there is always the temptation to use a search engine and read only the first study that comes up; this would not only be lazy, but risky.

The World Health Organization declared the coronavirus (Covid-19) to be a pandemic on 12 March 2020. There was a need for much new research into the control and treatment of Covid-19; but there was also a need to have a good understanding about what was already known. Wasting valuable time and resources on replicating existing knowledge is not acceptable in any circumstances, least of all in this situation. Already by 6 April 2020, one of the main control measures, that of school closures, was critically examined in a rapid systematic review of school closures and other school social distancing practices across the world [1]. Such a review is far more useful to policy-makers and the public than looking at original studies, many of which will be behind paywalls and so inaccessible to most people and who also may not understand the methodological and statistical details of the papers

© The Editor(s) (if applicable) and The Author(s), under exclusive license to Springer Nature Switzerland AG 2020
E. Purssell, N. McCrae, *How to Perform a Systematic Literature Review*,
https://doi.org/10.1007/978-3-030-49672-2_1

even if they did have the time and inclination to read them all. This is the role of the systematic review.

One example of what can go wrong, with devastating consequences, was with the measles, mumps, and rubella (MMR) vaccine. One ill-judged case series that suggested a link between the MMR vaccine and autism, subsequently retracted [2], was the basis for a rumour that reduced public confidence in the vaccine to such an extent that many parents refused to have their children vaccinated. As a result of this, we saw epidemics of diseases in places where they were thought well controlled. Had people been able to look not just at the one study but the entire body of literature the lack of evidence for this association, this might have been avoided. Actually, the work of the reviewer entails looking critically at the literature, in this case recognising the inherent weaknesses of the case series as a form of evidence and other clues perhaps to the veracity of any claims [3]. In pointing this out, we are not saying that the case series is a flawed methodology, just that it can never show cause and effect. To see the correct use of a case series like this, we might look at a paper in the American Morbidity and Mortality Weekly Report from 1981, which reported the cases of five apparently healthy young men with *Pneumocystis* pneumonia. This was interesting because this condition is very unusual, and to see so many cases in apparently healthy people was unknown. We now know that they were the first reported cases of acquired immune deficiency syndrome (AIDS). However, starting the findings, the conclusion though is appropriately measured: 'All the above observations suggest the possibility of a cellular-immune dysfunction related to a common exposure that predisposes individuals to opportunistic infections such as pneumocystosis and candidiasis' [4].

Because they use the entire body of literature, systematic reviews are widely regarded as the highest form of evidence by the scientific community. Rigour and replication are the bedrocks of science. In this regard, review methodologies have undergone enormous change in recent years, indeed during the period over which this book has written new tools and techniques have become available. The days of a systematic review being comprised of a few papers you have hanging around plus a quick search are long gone! As we emphasise throughout this book, a review should produce a whole greater than the sum of parts. Whether the reviewed studies are quantitative or qualitative, the output is more than a summary; a distinct contribution to knowledge is made by interpreting the weight and meaning of evidence.

The above requirements mean that writing a systematic review requires a team that usually encompasses subject experts, at least one person who is knowledgeable about literature search strategies, systematic review methodologists, someone experienced in the methods used to analyse the data and a team to write the review. Our own contributions to the systematic review literature have encompassed mental health [5, 6], infection control [7] and child health [8, 9].

It is important to stress that systematic reviews cannot be conducted on every topic, and in some areas, it is more difficult than others. It relies on the question being amenable to research; not all are. It relies on literature being available. It also relies on a sensitivity to and understanding of the difficulties of the primary researchers. Research can be a long, frustrating and lonely business; reviewers should always remember this when reviewing the work of others.

For budding systematic reviewers, we hope that this book will inform and inspire you. We also hope that it helps experienced reviewers and academic supervisors to reconsider some of their assumptions. We are all learning all of the time, and this book is certainly not the last word, but we are confident that our guidance will keep you on the right track, heading in the right direction.

1.1 How to Read This Book

Although a systematic review has distinct parts, they only really make sense as a whole; one part informs the next. We suggest that you read each chapter as you go along. Each chapter can be used individually, but it may require some flicking back and forth between chapters. We have indicated in the text where this may be needed.

All of the references are in a Zotero Group; you can access this here: https://www.zotero.org/groups/2460528/systematicreviewbook/items/APGI5B9K/library.

Acknowledgements We would like to acknowledge all of those who have helped through education and experience in our development as nurses and scholars. In particular, Edward would like to thank Jeannine who has put up with so much and the staff and students at King's College London and more recently City, University of London, alongside whom he has polished his reviewing skills. Niall would like to thank Catherine and the girls and all those who have supported him through thick and thin.

References

1. Viner RM, Russell SJ, Croker H et al (2020) School closure and management practices during coronavirus outbreaks including COVID-19: a rapid systematic review. Lancet Child Adolesc Health 4:397–404. https://doi.org/10.1016/S2352-4642(20)30095-X
2. Wakefield A, Murch S, Anthony A et al (1998) RETRACTED: Ileal-lymphoid-nodular hyperplasia, non-specific colitis, and pervasive developmental disorder in children. Lancet 351:637–641. https://doi.org/10.1016/S0140-6736(97)11096-0
3. Deer B (2011) How the case against the MMR vaccine was fixed. BMJ 342:c5347. https://doi.org/10.1136/bmj.c5347
4. MMWR (1981) Pneumocystis pneumonia—Los Angeles. https://www.cdc.gov/mmwr/preview/mmwrhtml/june_5.htm. Accessed 15 Apr 2020
5. Keles B, McCrae N, Grealish A (2020) A systematic review: the influence of social media on depression, anxiety and psychological distress in adolescents. Int J Adolesc Youth 25:79–93. https://doi.org/10.1080/02673843.2019.1590851
6. McCrae N, Gettings S, Purssell E (2017) Social media and depressive symptoms in childhood and adolescence: a systematic review. Adolesc Res Rev 2:315–330. https://doi.org/10.1007/s40894-017-0053-4
7. Purssell E, Gould D, Chudleigh J (2020) Impact of isolation on hospitalised patients who are infectious: systematic review with meta-analysis. BMJ Open 10:e030371. https://doi.org/10.1136/bmjopen-2019-030371

8. Bertille N, Purssell E, Hjelm N et al (2018) Symptomatic management of febrile illnesses in children: a systematic review and meta-analysis of parents' knowledge and behaviors and their evolution over time. Front Pediatr 6:279. https://doi.org/10.3389/fped.2018.00279
9. Purssell E, Collin J (2016) Fever phobia: the impact of time and mortality—a systematic review and meta-analysis. Int J Nurs Stud 56:81–89. https://doi.org/10.1016/j.ijnurstu.2015.11.001

A Brief History of the Systematic Review

2

Summary Learning Points

- The concept of evidence-based practice is not new, but it has been inconsistently applied in practice.
- Systematic review methodologies have developed over time and will continue to do so. This means that reviews conducted some years ago will often have different reporting and methodological qualities to those done today.
- Review methodology changes frequently, and it is important that those teaching and conducting them stay up to date with current practices.
- Systematic reviews should be treated as any other kind of research, and it is important to recognise their limitations as well as their strengths and to be measured when making claims of causation.

2.1 Literature Past and Present

Let us contrast nursing and medicine in how they read research. Most nurses in current practice received their education at university, having entered the professional register with a degree. Until the late twentieth century, however, nurses were trained in a hospital-based school of nursing, near the wards and their living quarters (in some hospitals, the school occupied the ground floor of the nurses' home). Traditionally, training was an apprenticeship, with little academic demand. Recruits had chosen a practical discipline—and discipline it was, with strictly enforced rituals and routine. In a gendered division of labour, the good (female) nurse was neatly groomed, diligent and obedient to (male) doctors.

Examinations and essays during training were handwritten, with no requirement for references. The library of a typical school of nursing held collections of the weekly *Nursing Times* and *Nursing Mirror* magazines, alongside standard textbooks on anatomy and various fields of nursing practice. Controversy was scarce, because all nursing schools provided the same information, and uncertainty about diagnoses or treatments was rarely debated. Instead of the multidisciplinary ethos of today, most reading material was specifically for nurses, and nursing knowledge was

© The Editor(s) (if applicable) and The Author(s), under exclusive license to Springer
Nature Switzerland AG 2020
E. Purssell, N. McCrae, *How to Perform a Systematic Literature Review*,
https://doi.org/10.1007/978-3-030-49672-2_2

predominantly about care rather than treatment. Consequently, nursing students and fledgling nursing researchers learned to make do with a limited array of literature. To some extent, this disciplinary isolation persists in the notion of 'nursing research methods'.

Medical libraries were on a higher academic plane. Trainees delved into peer-reviewed journals, which filled the shelves from floor to ceiling. Annual volumes of the *Lancet*, *British Medical Journal* and a plethora of specialist publications were collated in bespoke binders; new editions were placed on a rack for ready access. Whereas books were soon outdated, journals presented the latest available research findings (albeit months after the authors had completed their study). Three or four decades ago, there were considerably fewer journals, and it was possible for trainees or researchers in better-endowed medical schools to complete a fairly thorough literature review over a few days in the library. Indexes of literature existed in the predigital era but were cumbersome and infrequently updated. Writers often relied on reference lists to find relevant papers. Interlibrary arrangements enabled retrieval of papers from journals held elsewhere, but there was often a long wait for photocopies from elusive sources.

Students have less need to visit a library today. Paper copies are no longer published by most journals, and the accumulated binders from earlier decades have disappeared from the modern electronic library, which mostly exists in virtual form on an intranet. Literature searches are automated, using bibliographic databases such as Medline. However, not all universities have the same resources, as online journal and database subscriptions are expensive (like pubs that show live football matches, libraries pay much higher fees than charged to an individual subscriber). To use cable television as an analogy, the premier seats of learning, such as the Russell Group universities in the UK or the Ivy League in the USA, purchase the full package with movies and live football, while the former polytechnic colleges are restricted to news channels, soap operas and quiz shows.

Meanwhile, the academic publishing system is changing radically. Increasingly authors are paying for readers to have open access to their papers, thereby maximising readership and impact. Sooner rather than later, this will become the only way to get published in journals. Healthcare knowledge is apparently being liberalised, but there are pitfalls in this progressive venture. The typical fee of around £2000 ($2500) should be included in the study funding application. Fees are likely to increase after the current transitional phase, as academic publishers will depend on researchers for income. However, not all studies are funded. Consequently, small-scale qualitative studies, which can be useful primers for more substantial research, might be inhibited. Literature reviews, which may be a product of students' dissertations or ad hoc projects by faculty staff, could also be curtailed by publication costs. Nursing has tended to receive a smaller 'slice of the cake' in research funding, and the new business model could perpetuate power imbalance towards privileged institutions and professions.

The peer-reviewing model continues as before, but a growing number of journals are competing for a limited pool of expert reviewers. Business interests might influence publishing decisions: journals need papers to survive. There is danger of quantity undermining quality, as new or obscure journals offer novice writers certainty of publication (for a price). As soon as a writer gains a publication record, he or she will be bombarded with unsolicited requests from predatory journals to submit a paper. Unwary readers who stumble across this terrain are exposed to poorly conducted and inadequately reviewed studies. Many of these titles will not be indexed by research databases. In their pursuit of evidence from all valid sources, literature reviewers should be aware of these trends in publishing and any inherent loss of quality control or bias.

Literature reviewing is in some ways easier and in other ways more challenging than in the past. Everything now is digital and increasingly accessible. The process of reviewing has developed, with established rules for performing and reporting. Scientific standards have been raised in the form of the systematic literature review, which has become the prime information resource for healthcare practitioners. However, a plethora of tools and checklists might seem more of a hindrance than a help.

2.2   A Man with a Mission

Although he was not the first to call for a stronger scientific basis to healthcare, Archibald (Archie) Cochrane is justly honoured as the architect of evidence-based practice, and his life story is worth telling. Born in Galashiels, Scotland, in 1909, Cochrane had porphyria at birth, a condition that influenced his professional career [1]. Gaining a place at the University of Cambridge, on graduation in 1931, he became a research student in a tissue culture laboratory. Dissatisfied with this work, he moved to Germany to study psychoanalysis under Theodor Reik, who had been one of Sigmund Freud's first students. Reik fled persecution by the Nazi regime, and Cochrane followed him to Vienna and then to the Netherlands. In his own analysis by Reik, Cochrane discussed a sexual problem that he attributed to his porphyria. However, he derived little benefit from such therapy, and he concluded that psychoanalysis lacked scientific basis.

Cochrane began medical training, which was interrupted by the Second World War. He enlisted but was captured in action by the Germans. As a prisoner of war, his modest grasp of German language and his medical proficiency gained him a dual appointment as medical officer and negotiator. He conducted a dietary trial and persuaded the camp administrators that a yeast supplement would cure the widespread problem of oedema among inmates. After the war, he completed his training at the University College Hospital in London and undertook specialist training in epidemiology, an emerging branch of medical science that explores the causes of disease by statistical rather than laboratory methods. Cochrane worked in a research unit on pneumoconiosis, which was a particular health hazard in the massive workforce of coal miners. This led to a professorship of tuberculosis in Wales. He was also appointed as honorary director of the Medical Research Council Epidemiology Unit, where he introduced a grading scale for response rates in studies (a rate of 91% scored 1 'Cochrane units', 95% scored 2 units; less than 90% was deemed unacceptable).

Awarded a fellowship by the Nuffield Provincial Hospitals Trust, Cochrane wrote an incisive review of the National Health Service (NHS). His short monograph *Effectiveness and Efficiency* [2] applied three measures: effectiveness (whether a treatment changes the course of a disease), efficiency (how well the NHS deployed resources such as staff and equipment to deliver an intervention) and equality (consistency of access to care and variation between hospitals). Cochrane was scathing of NHS medicine for its untested treatments and unfounded assumptions in clinical practice. Tonsillectomy, for example, was very frequently performed on children, but often without clear indication. Overtreatment entailed unnecessary hospital admission and surgery. By contrast, other medical conditions were undertreated, particularly in the elderly. Variation in care may be justified by individual patient's circumstances, but not by institutional discrimination.

Cochrane promoted randomised controlled trials (RCT) as the best evidence for any treatment. However, research often produced contrary results, as with the outcomes of tonsillectomy, and practitioners were unsure about which findings had most weight. Cochrane [3] remarked: 'It is surely a great criticism of our profession that we have not organised a critical summary, by specialty or subspecialty, adapted periodically, of all relevant randomised controlled trials'. By instilling a rigorous approach to understanding and applying empirical evidence, Cochrane's legacy was to integrate research and practice. By the turn of the millennium, the doctrine of evidence-based medicine was firmly established [4].

2.3   Hierarchy of Evidence

By the time of Cochrane's call for better evidence, the RCT had been in use in medical research for some decades. Experimental methodology was the vehicle for the tremendous growth of the pharmaceutical industry in the mid-twentieth century, as the marketing success of a new drug depended on convincing results. In clinical practice, however, prescribing by doctors was often based on untested assumptions. For example, until the 1950s, it was not unusual for patients suffering from anxiety or stress to be advised to smoke. The discovery of a causative link between smoking and lung cancer was a turning point in medicine, because it demonstrated the necessity for scientific investigation and evidence (although Cochrane himself was not deterred from his nicotine habit).

One of the most famous studies in the history of medical research was by Austin Bradford Hill and Richard Doll, who showed that smoking causes lung cancer. In 1947, the Medical Research Council (MRC) appointed a team of experts to investigate the troubling increase in incidence of this disease, and Bradford Hill was chosen following his work on tuberculosis, a wasting disease that had become known as the scourge of humankind. As a young man, Bradford Hill had been expected to follow his father's footsteps into medicine, but he was waylaid by tuberculosis [5]. There was no effective treatment, and like many thousands of other sufferers, he was sent to a sanitorium, where the disease was slowed by a regime of fresh air (beds were wheeled out to verandahs). Bradford Hill was treated by the surgical procedure of pneumothorax, whereby air was pumped into the pleural cavity to reduce the size of the lung and constrain the tubercles. For most patients, pneumothorax merely delayed their inevitable demise, but surprisingly, Bradford Hill made a full recovery.

After a correspondence course in economics, in the 1930s, Bradford Hill began his career in epidemiology. As professor of medical statistics at the London School of Hygiene and Tropical Medicine, in 1946, he led a study of streptomycin, a drug that had shown potential against the tubercle bacillus. Guiding Bradford Hill was the seminal work of statistician Ronald Fisher, whose *Statistical Methods for Research Workers* of 1925 emphasised significance testing of experimental results to assess the possibility of chance. Fisher's later book *The Design of Experiments* [6] asserted clinical trials and statistical analysis as the foundation for medical treatment.

Bradford Hill organised a randomised trial at three London hospitals, comparing 55 patients treated by streptomycin with 52 patients on the usual regime of bed rest. After 6 months, 28 in the streptomycin group had considerably improved; there had been 4 deaths compared with 14 in the control group. However, 3 years later, 32 of the treated group had died, showing that while streptomycin worked in the short term, the pathogen was resistant. Bradford Hill conducted another trial combining streptomycin and para-amino salicylic acid, and this raised the survival rate to over 80%. Tuberculosis was demonstrably curable, an achievement attributed to the rigour of the RCT.

With effective prevention and treatment, mortality from pulmonary tuberculosis declined. By 1950, it was overtaken by lung cancer. At the outset of their MRC lung cancer study, Doll and Bradford Hill did not suspect smoking as the carcinogenic culprit, thinking instead of environmental factors such as pollution from motor transport [5]. Their prospective cohort study of doctors on the British medical register produced seemingly irrefutable evidence of the carcinogenic effect of smoking: heavy smokers were more likely to succumb than light smokers, and doctors who never smoked were 40 times less likely to get lung cancer than those who smoked 25 or more cigarettes per day.

To study the effects of smoking, a randomised trial would not have been feasible, due to the high prevalence of the behaviour (in the 1950s, almost 90% of the adult population smoked) and the long time period necessary for assessing the outcome of interest (cancer). However, evidence from a case-control or cohort study is not as conclusive as that from an RCT, because other known or unknown factors could cause differences between groups. Correlation, we must remember, is not causation (for a while, many in the medical profession dismissed the results of Doll and Bradford Hill, suggesting confounding factors as the cause). Bradford Hill presented the following criteria for correlation in medical research: it must be biologically plausible, strong, consistent and preferably confirmed by experimental methods and show a gradient by exposure.

In 1962, the Federal Drug Administration in the USA required all new drugs to be tested by clinical trials in human beings. However, as with any research activity, RCTs do not guarantee robust evidence. Quality can vary in design and conduct, including sample size, attrition and the time period between baseline and outcome measurement. Furthermore, omissions in reporting could undermine the results, whatever the statistical or clinical significance. In 1993, a group of journal editors, clinical trialists and epidemiologists gathered in Ottawa, Canada, to develop a scale to assess the quality of RCT reporting. They produced a set of desirable items, many of which were inadequately reported in journals. Meanwhile a gathering in California, the Asilomar Research Group, devised another checklist. At the suggestion of the *Journal of the American Medical Association* editor Drummond Rennie, these two bodies convened in Chicago, and the outcome was the Consolidated Standards of Reporting Trials (CONSORT). The statement guided authors on essential information to be presented, enabling readers to judge the validity of study results [7]. A comparative evaluation [8] showed that CONSORT raised the quality of trials published in healthcare journals, not only in reporting but also in the conduct of research (although the latter was not directly covered by the statement). The statement was revised in 2001 and 2010.

In 1989, David Sackett, clinical epidemiologist at McMaster University in Canada, proposed a grading of recommendations from studies of antithrombotic agents. RCTs were placed first (subdivided into trials with large and small effect size), followed by cohort and case-control studies, case series and lastly expert opinion and anecdotal experience [9]. In 1994, Sackett was invited to lead the new Oxford Centre for Evidence-Based Medicine, and with Gordon Guyatt and others, he presented the first generic hierarchy of evidence for biomedical research [10], which healthcare evaluation expert Greenhalgh [11] reconfigured in the following order:

1. Systematic reviews/meta-analyses of RCTs
2. RCTs with definitive results
3. RCTs without definitive results
4. Cohort studies
5. Case-control studies
6. Cross-sectional surveys
7. Case series

The significant development here is that the hierarchy is topped not by primary research but by the secondary activity of reviewing research.

2.4   The Rise of the Systematic Review

By the late twentieth century, it was becoming very difficult for busy clinicians to know the best and latest evidence to guide practice. The problem was not only the overwhelming amount of literature but also the variable quality of reviewing. Examining 50 review papers in leading medical journals, Mulrow [12] found that almost all were 'subjective, scientifically unsound, and inefficient'. Having scrutinised 83 meta-analyses of RCTs, Sacks and colleagues [13] urged a more robust approach to searching, evaluating and synthesising evidence. A similar investigation of 36 reviews in medical journals by Oxman and Guyatt [14] came to the unflattering conclusion 'that experts, on average, write reviews of inferior quality; that the greater the expertise the more likely the quality is to be poor; and that the poor quality may be related to the strength of the prior opinions and the amount of time they spend preparing a review article'.

In 1993, 5 years after Archie Cochrane died, the Cochrane Collaboration was founded by Chalmers [15], with the practical aim of informing clinical practice by conducting and disseminating systematic reviews of medical interventions. The Cochrane Collaboration produced a manual for systematic reviewing, which has been regularly updated. According to the *Cochrane Handbook for Systematic Reviews of Interventions* [16], a systematic review has the following features:

- Clearly stated set of objectives with a priori eligibility criteria
- Explicit, reproducible method
- Comprehensive search that attempts to find all eligible studies
- Assessment of validity of the included studies (e.g. risk of bias)
- Systematic presentation and synthesis of the findings of included studies

Therefore, while the traditional literature review is a discursive text that may give subjective prominence to the most interesting or influential studies, the systematic review is an objective and standardised exercise. The Centre for Reviews and Dissemination, founded in 1994 at the University of York with government funding to conduct and collate systematic reviews in healthcare, issued the following definition [17]:

> A review of the evidence on a clearly formulated question that uses systematic and explicit methods to identify, select and critically appraise relevant primary research, and to extract and analyse data from the studies that are included in the review.

The term 'meta-analysis' was introduced by Glass [18] of Arizona State University for combining the results of multiple studies. An early exemplar in medicine was a meta-analysis of 25 trials of antiplatelet treatment [19], which comprised a total of over 29,000 patients with a history of transient ischaemic attacks, occlusive strokes, unstable angina or myocardial infarction. Meta-analysis produces a more precise estimate of an effect size and is particularly useful for showing rare events, which might be missed by single studies of limited statistical power. Although synonymous with 'systematic review' in American journals, in European journals, 'meta-analysis' is reserved for reviews that statistically analyse data from studies (see Chap. 6). Whether or not such analysis is performed, a systematic review is an original report of research evidence with interpretation and recommendations, amounting to a whole greater than the sum of parts [20].

The Cochrane Library is a valuable repository of systematic reviews to inform practice. Other bodies publish treatment recommendations based on reviews of research. In the UK, the National Institute for Health and Care Excellence (NICE) produces clinical guidelines for a growing number of health conditions. Founded in 1999 by the government, the NICE was intended to improve consistency of healthcare throughout the NHS. Its reviews take into account medical and economic factors while also considering patients' perspectives. For example, NICE guidelines on depression [21] emphasise the individual patient's preference for antidepressant drugs or talking therapy. Another example is the guidelines produced by the Canadian Nurses Association [22], based on research evidence and clinical consensus in nursing activities such as pain management.

Systematic reviews present a critical summary of evidence, but readers should always consider the possibility of bias or other anomalies, whoever the author or whatever the journal. Just as quality standards were instilled for reporting of RCTs, systematic reviewers are expected to demonstrate rigour. In 1996, an international group of 30 epidemiologists, researchers, journal editors, statisticians and clinicians devised the Quality of Reporting of Meta-Analyses (QUORUM) checklist, to ensure consistency and transparency in reviews of RCTs. In 2009, the guidelines were revised with an expanded scope and were renamed Preferred Reporting Items for Systematic Reviews and Meta-Analyses (PRISMA) [23]. A cardinal feature of PRISMA is a flowchart showing the progression from initial search result through a screening process to the ultimately included studies (see Chap. 4). Most health science journals have endorsed PRISMA as a reporting requirement for reviewers.

2.5   Numbers Are Not Enough

Having initially focussed on RCTs, the systematic review dealt with studies of standardised design and reporting. However, the experimental method is not always appropriate in providing answers to human problems. Moreover, the meaning of literature is not always quantifiable. The ascent of evidence-based medicine, with its apparent fixation on trials and systematic reviews, spurred dissent within the profession. Critics argued that the favoured hierarchy of evidence was simplistic, that it encouraged instrumentalism and impeded individualised care and that it had been hijacked by the pharmaceutical industry. Evidence-based medicine is normative, but not a philosophical framework [24]. However, a knowledge system that values scientific evidence is not necessarily reductionist. Sackett and colleagues [25] defined evidence-based medicine as 'the conscientious, explicit and judicious use of current best evidence in making decisions about the care of individual patients'. Treatment, therefore, should be decided by professional judgement, informed rather than imposed by research findings.

Since the 1990s, a more inclusive approach to evidence has emerged, as the original concept of evidence-based medicine was renamed 'evidence-based practice'. A high proportion of medical interventions have never been tested by RCTs, and this is more so in other disciplines such as nursing and social work. Drug treatments are amenable to experimental investigation, with sampling and statistical analysis fixed on a primary outcome variable, but the limits of an exclusively RCT-based systematic review are exposed in the context of complex interventions. For example, in an evaluation of postgraduate medical education, Greenhalgh and colleagues [26] found merely one RCT, which would have severely limited the validity of the review.

Another body promoting research evidence was founded in the name of American social psychologist Donald T. Campbell. In the 1960s, Campbell led major evaluations of federal welfare programmes in the USA. Author of the book *Experimental and Quasi-Experimental Designs for Research*, which became the 'bible' for evaluating social policy, Campbell envisaged a socially engineered world in which every problem was amenable to solutions based on scientific evidence. He described government reforms as societal experiments, at a time when social and psychological sciences were dominated by behaviourism and the pursuit of predictive laws of human behaviour. However, Campbell realised that testing of stimulus-response mechanisms was unsuitable for social interventions, which defied the precision of variables and measurement required for RCTs. Evaluations of experimental design failed to deliver the desired explanatory information; evidence was narrow if not spurious and consequently of limited use to decision-makers. Based on his wealth of experience, Campbell developed a meta-methodological approach to evaluation [27], emphasising process as well as outcomes. He is regarded as one of the most influential social scientists. In 2000, following a meeting of social and behavioural scientists at the University College London, including several members of the Cochrane Collaboration, the Campbell Collaboration was founded to evaluate social science policy.

Debate about reductionism is particularly relevant to nursing research, with its qualitative tradition. There is tension, often unacknowledged in nurse education, between the potentially conflicting doctrines of evidence-based practice and person-centred care [28]. A sophisticated approach is necessary in generating evidence and in interpreting and applying the results of research. As French [29] argued, evidence-based practice in nursing makes use of tacit, experiential knowledge in tandem with generic theory and evidence. Carper [30] formulated four ways of knowing in nursing practice:

- Empirics (verifiable, objective knowledge)
- Aesthetics (tacit, intuitive)
- Ethics (moral)
- Personal knowing (unique perspectives formed by character and experience)

A systematic review is primarily concerned with the first of these ways of knowing. Nursing is an applied science, and empirical evidence is crucial: some interventions have stronger evidence than others, while there are potential costs as well as benefits. Back in the nineteenth century, Florence Nightingale collated statistics on morbidity and mortality, comparing hospitals and districts. She revealed areas of concern and showed what could be achieved by better care [31]. Founder of the modern nursing profession, Nightingale was a pioneer of evidence-based practice, but she would have known that numbers are never enough [32]. Experience counts too.

Empirical evidence is not restricted to quantitative study results. The findings of a qualitative study are also the product of scientific investigation. Anecdote is not the singular of data. Qualitative research does more than collect individual accounts; it interprets as well as describes. Not long ago, qualitative methods lacked credibility in medicine, where 'hard' evidence was expected. This changed not only due to improvements in qualitative methods but also emancipatory social forces and acceptance that science cannot truly explain if it ignores human experience. Epistemology (how we can know reality) has broadened in the health disciplines to include interpretative analysis of patients and practitioners' perspectives, alongside the conventional scientific activities of trials and cohort studies. However, the *BMJ* [33] recently caused a stir by declaring that it would prioritise research with definitive results over exploratory findings, thereby eschewing qualitative studies. Greenhalgh and colleagues [34] criticised this decision for stifling the type of research that shows 'why promising clinical interventions do not always work in the real world, how patients experience care, and how practitioners think'.

Qualitative research has been neglected in systematic literature reviewing. In an editorial in the *International Journal of Nursing Studies* (the world's leading nursing journal by impact factor), Norman and Griffiths [35] expressed concern that literature reviews were becoming too formulaic, adhering to a narrow procedure appropriate for RCTs but not other types of study:

> There appears to be a growing belief that a review is not worth reading unless it is a systematic review. This, we contend, is simply not true.

Not all reviews, they asserted, should be of the systematic type. For example, a literature review for a doctoral thesis has a broader, scholarly purpose, exploring knowledge on relevant theory and concepts and telling a story rather than summarising evidence on cause-and-effect variables. Indeed, the narrative review is the 'bread and butter' of a liberal university education, as it entails critical reasoning to develop a coherent argument. The novice reviewer should be alert to such differences in choosing and following textbooks. For example, Hart's [36] *Doing a Literature Review* is a guide to the narrative form of review in social science, as is Ridley's [37] *The Literature Review: A Step-by-Step Guide for Students* (although the back cover states that this book 'describes how to carry out a literature review in a systematic, methodical way'). Another type is the scoping review, which examines what is known about a topic, including policy document and expert opinion as well as studies. Metasynthesis, as described by Griffiths and Norman [38], is the qualitative version of a systematic review (see Chap. 7).

For Polit and Beck [39], authors of a popular text on nursing research, a systematic review may cover any or all types of research methods, including quantitative, qualitative and mixed-method studies. In 1996, a global collaboration of scientists and practitioners was founded at the University of Adelaide in Australia, with a pragmatist orientation to promoting evidence-based practice. The Joanna Briggs Institute, named after the first matron of the Royal Adelaide Hospital, provides guidance and tools for reviewing literature of mixed research methodology, helping reviewers to synthesise different types of evidence. As Greenhalgh [40] argues, to understand what works in healthcare, the horizon should be broadened to encompass process as well as outcomes. This makes literature reviewing more challenging, but also more truthful.

2.6 Conclusion

As research methods have diversified, so has the scope of literature reviewing. There are various ways to describe and critically analyse literature, but a properly conducted and reported systematic review offers the most robust evidence for clinical practice. Rigour must go hand in hand with relevance. Healthcare reviewers should never lose sight of their *raison d'être*, which is to contribute to practical knowledge, informing practitioners, patients, policy-makers and the public.

References

1. Shah HM, Chung KC (2009) Archie Cochrane and his vision for evidence-based medicine. Plast Reconstr Surg 124:982–988. https://doi.org/10.1097/PRS.0b013e3181b03928
2. Cochrane AL (1972) Effectiveness and efficiency: random reflections on health services. Nuffield Provincial Hospitals Trust, London
3. Cochrane A (1979) 1931–1971: a critical review, with particular reference to the medical profession. In: Medicines for the year 2000. Office of Health Economics, London
4. Djulbegovic B, Guyatt GH (2017) Progress in evidence-based medicine: a quarter century on. Lancet 390:415–423. https://doi.org/10.1016/S0140-6736(16)31592-6
5. Le Fanu J (2011) The rise & fall of modern medicine. Abacus, London
6. Fisher RA (1935) Design of experiments. Oliver and Boyd, Oxford
7. Begg C (1996) Improving the quality of reporting of randomized controlled trials. The CONSORT statement. JAMA 276:637–639. https://doi.org/10.1001/jama.276.8.637
8. Moher D, Jones A, Lepage L, for the CONSORT Group (2001) Use of the CONSORT statement and quality of reports of randomized trials: a comparative before-and-after evaluation. JAMA 285:1992. https://doi.org/10.1001/jama.285.15.1992
9. Sackett DL (1989) Rules of evidence and clinical recommendations on the use of antithrombotic agents. Chest 95:2S–4S
10. Guyatt GH, Sackett DL, Sinclair JC et al (1995) Users' guides to the medical literature. IX. A method for grading health care recommendations. Evidence-Based Medicine Working Group. JAMA 274:1800–1804. https://doi.org/10.1001/jama.274.22.1800
11. Greenhalgh T (1997) How to read a paper : getting your bearings (deciding what the paper is about). BMJ 315:243–246. https://doi.org/10.1136/bmj.315.7102.243
12. Mulrow CD (1987) The medical review article: state of the science. Ann Intern Med 106:485–488. https://doi.org/10.7326/0003-4819-106-3-485
13. Sacks HS, Berrier J, Reitman D et al (1987) Meta-analyses of randomized controlled trials. N Engl J Med 316:450–455. https://doi.org/10.1056/NEJM198702193160806
14. Oxman AD, Guyatt GH (1993) The science of reviewing research. Ann N Y Acad Sci 703:125–133; discussion 133–134. https://doi.org/10.1111/j.1749-6632.1993.tb26342.x

15. Chalmers I (1993) The Cochrane collaboration: preparing, maintaining, and disseminating systematic reviews of the effects of health care. Ann N Y Acad Sci 703:156–163; discussion 163–165. https://doi.org/10.1111/j.1749-6632.1993.tb26345.x

16. McKenzie JE, Brennan SE, Ryan RE , Thomson HJ, Johnston RV, Thomas J (2019) Chapter 3: Defining the criteria for including studies and how they will be grouped for the synthesis. In: Higgins JPT, Thomas J, Chandler J, Cumpston M, Li T, Page MJ, Welch VA (eds). Cochrane Handbook for Systematic Reviews of Interventions version 6.0. (updated July 2019). Cochrane. https://www.training.cochrane.org/handbook

17. Centre for Reviews and Dissemination (ed) (2009) CRD's guidance for undertaking reviews in healthcare, 3rd edn. York Publishing Services, York

18. Glass GV (1976) Primary, secondary, and meta-analysis of research. Educ Res 5:3–8. https://doi.org/10.3102/0013189X005010003

19. Antiplatelet Trialists' Collaboration (1988) Secondary prevention of vascular disease by prolonged antiplatelet treatment. BMJ 296:320–331. https://doi.org/10.1136/bmj.296.6618.320

20. Olsson C, Ringnér A, Borglin G (2014) Including systematic reviews in PhD programmes and candidatures in nursing—"Hobson's choice"? Nurse Educ Pract 14:102–105. https://doi.org/10.1016/j.nepr.2014.01.005

21. National Institute for Health and Care Excellence (2009) Overview—Depression in adults: recognition and management—Guidance—NICE. https://www.nice.org.uk/guidance/cg90. Accessed 17 Apr 2020

22. Canadian Nurses Association (2010) Evidence-informed decision making and nursing practice. In: Evidence-informed decision making and nursing practice. https://www.cna-aiic.ca/en/nursing-practice/evidence-based-practice

23. Moher D, Liberati A, Tetzlaff J et al (2009) Preferred reporting items for systematic reviews and meta-analyses: the PRISMA statement. PLoS Med 6:e1000097. https://doi.org/10.1371/journal.pmed.1000097

24. Sehon SR, Stanley DE (2003) A philosophical analysis of the evidence-based medicine debate. BMC Health Serv Res 3:14. https://doi.org/10.1186/1472-6963-3-14

25. Sackett DL, Rosenberg WMC, Gray JAM et al (1996) Evidence based medicine: what it is and what it isn't. BMJ 312:71–72. https://doi.org/10.1136/bmj.312.7023.71

26. Greenhalgh T, Toon P, Russell J et al (2003) Transferability of principles of evidence based medicine to improve educational quality: systematic review and case study of an online course in primary health care. BMJ 326:142–145. https://doi.org/10.1136/bmj.326.7381.142

27. Campbell DT, Stanley JC (1966) Experimental and quasi-experimental designs for research, 2. Reprinted from "Handbook of research on teaching". Houghton Mifflin Comp., Boston, MA. Reprint. ISBN: 978-0-395-30787-2

28. McCrae N (2012) Evidence-based practice: for better or worse. Int J Nurs Stud 49:1051–1053. https://doi.org/10.1016/j.ijnurstu.2012.08.010

29. French P (1999) The development of evidence-based nursing. J Adv Nurs 29:72–78. https://doi.org/10.1046/j.1365-2648.1999.00865.x

30. Carper B (1978) Fundamental patterns of knowing in nursing. ANS Adv Nurs Sci 1:13–23. https://doi.org/10.1097/00012272-197810000-00004

31. Mackey A, Bassendowski S (2017) The history of evidence-based practice in nursing education and practice. J Prof Nurs 33:51–55. https://doi.org/10.1016/j.profnurs.2016.05.009

32. McDonald L (2001) Florence Nightingale and the early origins of evidence-based nursing. Evid Based Nurs 4:68–69. https://doi.org/10.1136/ebn.4.3.68

33. BMJ (2016) Is The BMJ the right journal for my research article?—The BMJ. https://www.bmj.com/about-bmj/resources-authors/bmj-right-journal-my-research-article. Accessed 17 Apr 2020

34. Greenhalgh T, Annandale E, Ashcroft R et al (2016) An open letter to The BMJ editors on qualitative research. BMJ 352:i563. https://doi.org/10.1136/bmj.i563

35. Norman I, Griffiths P (2014) The rise and rise of the systematic review. Int J Nurs Stud 51:1–3. https://doi.org/10.1016/j.ijnurstu.2013.10.014

36. Hart C (1998) Doing a literature review: releasing the social science research imagination. Sage Publications, London
37. Ridley D (2008) The literature review: a step-by-step guide for students. SAGE, London
38. Griffiths P, Norman I (2005) Science and art in reviewing literature. Int J Nurs Stud 42:373–376. https://doi.org/10.1016/j.ijnurstu.2005.02.001
39. Polit DF, Beck CT (2012) Nursing research: generating and assessing evidence for nursing practice, 9th edn. Wolters Kluwer Health/Lippincott Williams & Wilkins, Philadelphia, PA
40. Greenhalgh T (2018) How to implement evidence-based healthcare. Wiley, Hoboken, NJ

The Aim and Scope of a Systematic Review: A Logical Approach

3

Summary Learning Points
- A systematic literature review is a logical, linear process, where each part is informed by that preceding it.
- Several types of review question may be asked; common ones are those comparing interventions, diagnostic tests, prognostic factors or qualitative questions. The approach to each is slightly different, but the general principles remain the same.
- There are a number of standards that *must* be followed, as well as tools that *can* be used.
- Logical eligibility criteria are important, as if these are not correct, everything that follows will be incorrect as well. This is analogous to setting criteria for admitting participants to a study.

The essence of logical thinking may be demonstrated in answering the question: 'what determines the value of a house?' Generally, house prices have risen steadily in recent decades, although some reversals have occurred, for example, after the global financial crisis of 2008. There is much variation, with prices typically higher in major cities and lower in areas of industrial decline. Value depends not only on the physical size and features of the building but a plethora of extraneous factors: socio-economic wealth of the surrounding area, pleasantness of the environment, quality of schools and transport links. Yet this myriad can be reduced to a single variable. The answer to the question is simply stated in one word—'demand'. That is the power of logic.

Many studies are designed with a primary outcome measurement, and logic guides you in seeking the crucial information. Sometimes the novice reader of a study report cannot see the wood for the trees. In a typical abstract of a paper reporting a randomised trial of a drug, the results section may include numerous figures. There may be various results, each with P values or confidence intervals, but the overall treatment outcome might be overlooked. Statistical significance is important, but logically the trial is designed to compare, and we need to know the result

© The Editor(s) (if applicable) and The Author(s), under exclusive license to Springer Nature Switzerland AG 2020
E. Purssell, N. McCrae, *How to Perform a Systematic Literature Review*, https://doi.org/10.1007/978-3-030-49672-2_3

of that comparison. This relates to clinical significance: Is the difference observable and meaningful to practitioners and patients?

For an example of comparison, a drug intended to reduce obesity may be measured by body mass index (BMI). The single figure you should seek is the difference between experimental and control groups in outcome measurement. The same logic applies to a systematic review (and particularly a meta-analysis) of any treatment that is measured by the same variable across the included studies. Research questions in healthcare are not always so straightforward, but logical principles should always be applied.

3.1   Aim of a Review

Logic is necessary from the outset of a systematic review. What is it that you want to know? A review question, which presents the aim of the work, should be clearly focussed, enabling a disciplined enquiry rather than a trawl for interesting study results. Consider these two examples of review questions on the 'flu jab':

- What is known about the influenza vaccine in older people?
- What is the effectiveness of the influenza vaccine in older people?

The questions differ only in the term 'effectiveness', which makes the latter more suitable for a systematic literature review. The first question is broad, and it could be answered by including commentaries, policy documents and other types of publication, as well as empirical studies. It may tell the story of the development of vaccination for this common and sometimes dangerous malady.

The second question has distinct independent and dependent variables. The independent variable is the vaccine, and incidence or severity of influenza would be the dependent variable. In reviewing any intervention with an intended outcome, a neat configuration of the cause and effect should be presented. This is not always possible for a systematic review, which could include studies that measure numerous variables; sometimes the question may be exploratory. However, the more focussed, the better.

Take, for example, a review question 'what is the effectiveness of antidementia drugs?' Various types of information may be necessary in evaluating these drugs, including activities of daily living, mood, social activity, quality of life and carers' stress. However, one variable is likely to have prominence in the research, and this will relate to the intended purpose of the treatment. Antidementia drugs are primarily prescribed to maintain cognitive functioning [1]. Accordingly, a systematic review of these drugs may be to assess their performance on this variable. However, a review may instead focus on other variables, such as side effects. For inclusion, studies must produce results specific to the aim of the review.

An important consideration when proposing a literature review is whether this has been done before. Millions of papers are published in academic journals every year, and the healthcare literature continues to grow. Perhaps a review of your topic of interest was published 5 years ago. It is highly likely that new studies will have been published since then. Ideally, as recommended by the Cochrane Collaboration, a fresh review should match the design and conduct of the previous work. Regularly reviewing research is vital for updating evidence-based practice. If, however, a review was published less than a year ago, there may be little value in conducting another review on the same treatment and outcome.

To some readers, our emphasis on specificity may seem reductionist. Indeed, many healthcare interventions cannot be fully evaluated by statistical measurement on a single scale. However, a systematic reviewer does not necessarily attempt a comprehensive analysis. A concise review question, confined to clearly stated variables, prioritises rigour over breadth. A *proviso* is that the conclusion acknowledges the limits of the review, so that no claims are made beyond the scope of evidence.

3.2   PICO

Having established the primacy of the review question in a systematic review, let us make use of a helpful tool in determining this question. Anyone who has attended as much as an introductory lecture on systematic reviewing will know PICO, which is an acronym for four features of the studies pursued by a reviewer:

- Population: people with a disease or of a particular age or vulnerability
- Intervention: the treatment being studied
- Control: the comparison group (e.g. placebo or usual care)
- Outcome: the variable used to measure and compare the treatment and control groups

This formulation sets the scope of literature for a review, ensuring that the qualifying boundaries align with the stated aim. We find that students appreciate the orderliness of PICO. It is certainly a good structure for reviewing research on treatments, particularly for randomised controlled trials. However, often students find that their review topic does not readily fit this formulation. As educators, we sometimes see PICO tables with merely two rows filled (P and I or P and O), due to the lack of controlled studies or a single outcome. A review of the experiences of people with dementia, for example, will not have an intervention, a control or an outcome. Do not try to fit a square peg into a round hole. There is little value in presenting a PICO configuration if merely two of the letters apply. Utility may be broadened by changing the second letter from I to E, denoting exposure rather than intervention. Exposure is particularly relevant to epidemiological or qualitative research.

PRISMA and some other guidelines have extended the acronym to PICOS, with the additional letter denoting study type. The reviewer may decide to restrict a review of an intervention to randomised controlled trials or may allow any quantitative outcome studies. Other study designs may be sought, such as qualitative research. Normally it would be inappropriate to include literature reviews, because the material for your review should be original studies, not a second-hand account of these studies.

3.3   Types of Review Questions

Various types of question may be asked by a reviewer. The Cochrane Collaboration has a typology of three areas of enquiry: prognostic, diagnostic and interventional. Prognosis may include factors relating to outcomes of a health condition, not necessarily limited to people who are already sick. However, as it is generally understood to mean the course of disease, we have added a fourth category of epidemiological questions.

An epidemiological review could be a straightforward analysis of research on prevalence of a medical condition, or it could investigate the likelihood of contracting a disease. Aetiology is the study of causes of disease. However, a risk factor is not necessarily a presumed or putative cause, but is thought to be predictive of the disease. Risks may be direct or indirect. As aetiological research investigates exposure, the review will seek prospective cohort studies and possibly case-control and retrospective cohort studies. Here is a suggested PEO formulation for a review of smoking and lung cancer:

- Population: Adults in a particular district
- Exposure: Smoking (tobacco)
- Outcome: Lung cancer
- Study type: Cohort studies

A diagnostic review question typically asks whether an assessment procedure accurately identifies people with or without a condition, often compared to an established method. It is important that participants in studies are roughly similar in risk profile. Typically, the relevant research will comprise cross-sectional or cohort studies, although case-control studies might be conducted for a rare disease. Here is a PICO formulation for a diagnostic review question on human immunodeficiency virus (HIV) testing:

- Population: People with HIV
- Intervention: A new (fourth generation) antibody test
- Comparator: Currently used tests
- Diagnostic outcome: Sensitivity, specificity and positive/negative predictive value
- Study type: RCTs and quasi-experimental studies

Prognostic questions ask about the course of a disease: how it is likely to develop or the prospects of recovery. The best type of study for a prognostic question is a prospective cohort study, but case-control and retrospective cohort studies could also be used. Here is an example of a review of correlation between alcohol consumption and development of dementia in older people with mild cognitive impairment:

- Population: People with mild cognitive impairment
- Exposure: Alcohol
- Comparator exposure: No alcohol
- Prognostic outcome: Dementia
- Study type: Cohort or case-control studies

Intervention questions are the most common in systematic literature reviewing: What is the evidence for a particular treatment or process of care? The review will include studies that compare patients with or without the treatment of interest, and there is likely to be a primary outcome measurement (normally the intended purpose of the intervention).

Sometimes reviewers use the term 'effectiveness', although this may be a misnomer as it really means how a treatment works in practice, and many experimental studies are not designed for this. Consider a trial of a new drug for people with renal failure. The RCT will probably exclude people who are very sick, as they should receive the best available treatment rather than a new drug of unknown effect. If the study produces positive results, the first people likely to be offered this new treatment are the very sick people who were excluded from the research. The strength of RCTs is in their highly controlled design and conduct, but clinical practice is not so controllable. As RCTs assess efficacy (how a drug works in experimental conditions) but not effectiveness, quasi-experimental or cohort studies may be sought, depending on the review question.

Using the PICOS configuration, a review question to evaluate effectiveness of two analgesics following surgery would be framed as follows:

- Population: Postsurgical patients
- Intervention: Morphine plus ibuprofen
- Control: Morphine only
- Outcome: Pain
- Study type: RCTs

For reviews of topics studied qualitatively instead of quantitatively, PICO is inappropriate. A 'horses for courses' approach acknowledges that qualitative and quantitative paradigms are fundamentally different in how they generate knowledge. The SPIDER configuration [2] has broader latitude, potentially including subjective experiences as well as objectively measured outcomes. This acronym comprises sample, phenomenon of interest, design, evaluation and research type. Here is a suggested use of SPIDER for a review of the relationship between social media and depression in adolescents:

- Sample: Adolescents
- Phenomenon of interest: Social media use

- Design: Quasi-experimental, cohort, case-control or qualitative studies
- Evaluation: Depression
- Research type: Qualitative, quantitative or mixed-method

3.4   Eligibility Criteria

The scope of a systematic review should be set as concisely as possible, leaving minimal room for subjectivity. Criteria for selection are often described as 'inclusion and exclusion', but as we are encouraging logic, why use three words instead of one? The overarching term is 'eligibility'. Studies are either eligible or not, as decided by the reviewer's predetermined criteria. A priori demarcation of relevant research is as crucial to a systematic review as a hypothesis is to a clinical trial. The *Cochrane Handbook for Systematic Reviews* [3] stated:

> One of the features that distinguish a systematic review from a narrative review is the pre-specification of criteria for including and excluding studies.

Eligibility criteria must fit the logic of the review question. Here is an example of how erroneously vague or illogical criteria can undermine a reviewer's work. In a systematic review conducted by us [4], the question was whether the use of internet and social media influences depressive symptoms in adolescence. We needed to exclude any studies that selected younger people by existing mental health problems or excessive use of social media. To answer the question, we wanted studies with generic samples: participants who were chosen on the basis of age rather than by their status related to our independent or dependent variables. If we had included any study that targeted people known to be depressed, we would have distorted the findings of our review. In principle, such a study would have 100% prevalence—and 0% incidence!

According to the internationally approved PRISMA guidelines for reporting of systematic reviews [5], eligibility criteria should appear directly after the aims and objectives of the review. However, this is not always apparent in reviews published in academic journals. We investigated the quality of reporting of eligibility criteria in three prominent nursing journals, all of which endorse PRISMA reporting guidelines in their instructions for authors [6]. Our review (itself systematic) examined systematic reviews in the *International Journal of Nursing Studies* (*IJNS*), *Journal of Advanced Nursing* (*JAN*) and *Journal of Clinical Nursing* (*JCN*), over a period of 3 years. A total of 101 papers were included.

While adherence to PRISMA guidelines was generally evident, over three-quarters of reviewers placed eligibility criteria after the search procedure. This is illogical: you must state what you are looking for before you decide how you will look for it. In a few cases, inclusion and exclusion criteria were presented as a final stage of the screening process, indicating post hoc selection of search results. Such anomalies may have been a flaw in reporting rather than conduct, but they raise

Table 3.1 Placement of eligibility criteria in systematic reviews in nursing journals [6]

	Before search strategy	Amidst search strategy	After search strategy
IJNS (34)	16	1	17
JCN (31)	8	3	20
JAN (36)	0	2	34
Total (101)	24	6	71

Table 3.2 A student's draft inclusion and exclusion criteria

Inclusion criteria	Exclusion criteria
Dementia	Conditions other than dementia
Adults aged 65+	Adults aged <65, children
Experiences of people with dementia	Not studying experiences
Studies	Reviews, commentaries, policy documents
Qualitative methods/mixed methods	Quantitative methods with no qualitative data
In English language	Not in English language

doubts about the logical approach of the reviewers (Table 3.1). Consequently, this could undermine their results, as Berrios [7, pp. 20–21] explained:

> A posteriori selection or 'pruning' of information is to be discouraged, as it often introduces unacceptable biases (just as would happen if a researcher arbitrarily eliminated subjects from a project after they had met entry criteria).

3.5   Inclusion Versus Exclusion

An important consideration is the relationship between an inclusion and exclusion criterion: Is one simply the opposite of the other? Here is an example from a postgraduate student's draft review of studies exploring older persons' experiences of dementia (Table 3.2):

At first glance, this appears neat and orderly. The two sets of criteria are mutually exclusive. The student was following guidance in a popular guide to systematic reviewing by Aveyard [8]. So what is the problem?

We are about to use 'Occam's razor' on this student's work. This is named after William of Ockham (c1287–1347), a scholar at Oxford University, who asserted that wherever there are competing explanations, the simplest should be accepted until contrary evidence arises. A scientist should not present a tortuous reason for an outcome if a more obvious reason exists. This is parsimony, an enduring principle of science, and it should be applied in finding the most efficient and valid way to answer a research question. For a systematic review, eligibility criteria should be the most straightforward means of determining the literature to be reviewed.

Logicians analyse the validity of a statement by replacing concepts with symbols [9]. The left-side criteria in the student's table above represent 'A'; the other column is simply 'non-A'. Therefore, the whole right-side column in the table above could be discarded without any loss of information. If you seek studies of dementia, you don't need to declare that studies of other diseases will be excluded: the inclusion criterion is sufficient. Just as it is unnecessary to specify 'non-A', there is normally no need to specify diseases (e.g. diabetes mellitus, stroke) as exclusions: this would simply be excluding 'B' and 'C' when you have already limited your scope to 'A'.

To be fair, the student who prepared these eligibility criteria was following instruction in the manual he cited. Aveyard's guide [8, p. 76] gives the following example to guide the novice reviewer:

> Imagine you are doing a literature review exploring the effectiveness of a particular treatment or care intervention. Let's say your review question is, 'How effective are anti-bullying policies in preventing bullying behaviour in school age children?'
>
> Inclusion criteria: studies that explore the effectiveness of bullying policies
> Exclusion criteria: studies that explore aspects other than the effectiveness of bullying policies

Nursing students and researchers tend to follow what has been done before, as promulgated by lecturers, academic supervisors, dissertations, journals or textbooks. Presenting inclusion and exclusion criteria as oppositional seems to be a particular habit in nursing. A similar review of eligibility criteria that we conducted in three leading medical journals [10] showed various deviations from the PRISMA guidelines, but there were no cases of eligibility criteria presented in the form advised by Aveyard [8].

We shall make a radical statement here: a review with clear and comprehensive eligibility criteria does not need exclusions. The emphasis should be on what you want, rather than what you don't want. We are not proposing to banish exclusion criteria, but they should be used sparingly as qualifying conditions of the inclusion criteria. Instead of 'non-A', it should be 'A but'.

For example, in a review of studies of the experience of dementia in older people, the reviewer may not want studies that include certain types of dementia, e.g. Korsakow's syndrome (a condition attributed to chronic alcohol abuse). It would be sensible to specify this as an excluding criterion. Otherwise, it would need to be stated as negative in the inclusion criteria: 'dementia not Korsakow's'. Either is correct, but the former is a clearer expression, as shown below:

- *Inclusion criteria*
  - Dementia
  - Adults aged >65
  - Experiences of dementia
  - Empirical studies wholly or partly qualitative
- *Exclusion criterion*
  - Korsakow's syndrome

It is quite acceptable for a systematic reviewer to refine the review question and eligibility criteria after some initial searching. Often a very large amount of literature will encourage the reviewer to reduce the scope of review to make it more focussed and more manageable. However, this should be done for reasons of scientific rationale rather than convenience. In our aforementioned review of nursing journals, we found that many systematic reviewers restricted the literature in ways that seemed arbitrary. To avoid suspicion of subjective selection, logical decision-making should be displayed throughout the conduct and reporting of a review.

A common feature of systematic reviews in nursing journals is time restriction. Sometimes you see in magazines or websites a poll for the best songs or movies of all time. Typically, the results are skewed towards currently popular films or tunes, indicating a recency bias. In restricting studies to a recent time period, reviewers are also guilty of such bias but with more serious consequences. A review might misrepresent evidence by excluding older studies with important results. Rather than a deliberate manipulation of the literature, this is more likely to be a labour-saving device. A time restriction is typically justified as a pursuit of contemporary research, but this is not a scientifically valid concept. For example, a review question 'what is the evidence for anti-retroviral therapy in reducing mother-to-child transmission of human autoimmune virus?' restricted to the year 2000 onwards would neglect important early research, including a seminal study showing the effectiveness of zidovudine published in 1994 [11, 12]. A reviewer could legitimately exclude this study, but not merely because it is deemed too old.

In Aveyard's [8] glossary, the example given for inclusion criteria is 'research from the past 5 years'. In the text, Aveyard helpfully advises that 'if a pivotal event happened at a certain time that is relevant to your review, you might only be interested in literature published after that event' [8, p. 77]. However, this needs clarification for the novice reviewer. If a period is set, this must be justified. There is no need to set a time restriction at the introduction of a treatment, as there will be no research on that treatment before its existence.

Half of the papers in our investigation of systematic reviews in nursing journals had an unexplained or unsatisfactorily justified time restriction. In such reviews, the beginning of a search was typically set at the beginning of a decade (1970, 1980, 1990 or 2000) or a period of the last 10 years. Imagine a field of study that decided a 'year zero' for its literature: biology without Darwin, drama without Shakespeare, philosophy without Plato. In healthcare, it is nonsensical to include a paper published in January 2000 but not an equally valid study published in December 1999. Ad hoc restrictions are an unnecessary complication that divert from the logic of scientific enquiry (Fig. 3.1 and Table 3.3).

Similarly, many reviewers in our enquiry set arbitrary geographical limits. Unless there is a clear reason to do otherwise, a review should be comprehensive in coverage and therefore include relevant literature from anywhere in the world. Evidence is not normally specific to one county or region. To limit the scope to 'Western' healthcare systems is imprecise and could be politically contentious: Would Israel or Turkey, for example, be excluded? Research databases, as we will describe in the next chapter, have limitations in geographical and linguistic coverage, but there is no need to exacerbate the shortfall.

Related to geography is the use of language restrictions. Searching for studies reported in languages other than English potentially improves a systematic review

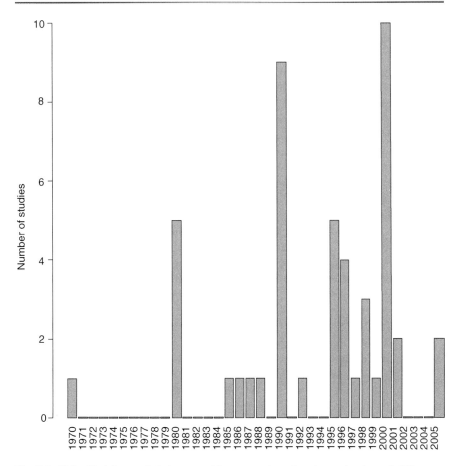

Fig. 3.1 Unjustified time periods (start year) in systematic reviews in nursing journals [6]

Table 3.3 Time restrictions in systematic reviews in nursing journals [6]

		Justification for time restriction		
Source and number of reviews	Number with time restriction	Satisfactory	Dubious	None
IJNS (34)	14	4	1	9
JCN (31)	20	2	4	14
JAN (36)	22	0	5	17
Total (101)	56	6	10	40

but is also challenging for the reviewer in obtaining and translating. Choice of languages often appeared arbitrary in our review of systematic reviews in nursing journals, apparently based on convenience (i.e. languages understood by members of the study team). A restriction to English, while biased, is generally acceptable due to the high proportion of journals published in this language. Reviewers may not be adding much value by including some but not all languages, unless this is a rational decision.

Table 3.4 'Dos and don'ts' for eligibility criteria

Topic of review	Inclusion	Exclusion	Comment
Cervical smear testing	Women	Men	Don't: Men obviously ineligible
		Pregnant	Do: Conditional eligibility
Depression in older people	Diagnosed depression	Dementia	Don't: If meant that study subjects have dementia instead of depression
		Comorbid dementia	Do: Conditional eligibility
Post-operative pain	Empirical studies	Commentary/ opinion articles	Don't: Unnecessary exclusion
	Empirical studies	Qualitative studies	Do: Conditional eligibility/ clarification
Effectiveness of ECT for depression	2000 onwards	–	Don't: Treatment was not changed at this time point
Impact of NICE guidelines for treatment of depression in the UK	2004 to present	–	Do: Studies will be irrelevant if published before the guidelines
Impact of Improving Access to Psychological Therapies (IAPT) scheme on employment	2006 to present	–	Don't: IAPT (a search term) did not exist before 2006 so no logical need for restriction

The need to include other languages depends on the review topic. A review of bacteriophage therapy for methicillin-resistant *Staphylococcus aureus* (MRSA) confined to papers in English would overlook extensive trials of this treatment reported in Russian journals [13]. A rapidly growing literature in Chinese languages may justify looking beyond the journals published in English, although many Oriental journals publish at least an abstract in English. If studies in other languages are not included, this should be stated as a limitation of the review.

As we have shown, some faulty habits have crept into systematic reviews in nursing. Here are some examples of useful and inappropriate exclusion criteria (Table 3.4):

For a fitting conclusion to this chapter, we shall borrow a dictum of psychologist Peterson [14], from his *Twelve Rules: An Antidote to Chaos*:

Do what is meaningful, not what is expedient.

References

1. O'Brien JT, Holmes C, Jones M et al (2017) Clinical practice with anti-dementia drugs: a revised (third) consensus statement from the British Association for Psychopharmacology. J Psychopharmacol (Oxford) 31:147–168. https://doi.org/10.1177/0269881116680924
2. Cooke A, Smith D, Booth A (2012) Beyond PICO: the SPIDER tool for qualitative evidence synthesis. Qual Health Res 22:1435–1443. https://doi.org/10.1177/1049732312452938

3. McKenzie JE, Brennan SE, Ryan RE, Thomson HJ, Johnston RV, Thomas J (2019) Chapter 3: Defining the criteria for including studies and how they will be grouped for the synthesis. In: Higgins JPT, Thomas J, Chandler J, Cumpston M, Li T, Page MJ, Welch VA (eds). Cochrane Handbook for Systematic Reviews of Interventions version 6.0 (updated July 2019), Cochrane. https://www.training.cochrane.org/handbook

4. McCrae N, Gettings S, Purssell E (2017) Social media and depressive symptoms in childhood and adolescence: a systematic review. Adolesc Res Rev 2:315–330. https://doi.org/10.1007/s40894-017-0053-4

5. Moher D, Liberati A, Tetzlaff J et al (2009) Preferred reporting items for systematic reviews and meta-analyses: the PRISMA statement. PLoS Med 6:e1000097. https://doi.org/10.1371/journal.pmed.1000097

6. McCrae N, Blackstock M, Purssell E (2015) Eligibility criteria in systematic reviews: a methodological review. Int J Nurs Stud 52:1269–1276. https://doi.org/10.1016/j.ijnurstu.2015.02.002

7. Berrios GE (1992) The review paper in psychiatry. In: Freeman C (ed) Research methods in psychiatry: a beginner's guide. 2nd rev. edn. Gaskell, London, pp 12–23

8. Aveyard H (2014) Doing a literature review in health and social care: a practical guide, 3rd edn. McGraw-Hill Education, Open University Press, Maidenhead

9. Hodges W (1977) Logic: an introduction to elementary logic. Penguin, Harmondsworth

10. McCrae N, Purssell E (2015) Eligibility criteria in systematic reviews published in prominent medical journals: a methodological review. J Eval Clin Pract 21:1052–1058. https://doi.org/10.1111/jep.12448

11. Connor EM, Sperling RS, Gelber R et al (1994) Reduction of maternal-infant transmission of human immunodeficiency virus type 1 with zidovudine treatment. N Engl J Med 331:1173–1180. https://doi.org/10.1056/NEJM199411033311801

12. Suksomboon N, Poolsup N, Ket-Aim S (2007) Systematic review of the efficacy of antiretroviral therapies for reducing the risk of mother-to-child transmission of HIV infection. J Clin Pharm Ther 32:293–311. https://doi.org/10.1111/j.1365-2710.2007.00825.x

13. Vlassov VV, Danishevskiy KD (2008) Biomedical journals and databases in Russia and Russian language in the former Soviet Union and beyond. Emerg Themes Epidemiol 5:15. https://doi.org/10.1186/1742-7622-5-15

14. Peterson JB, Doidge N (2018) 12 rules for life: an antidote to chaos. Allen Lane, London

Searching the Literature

4

Summary Learning Points
- Searching should follow a logical process but may be iterative as it sometimes takes more than one attempt to develop a search strategy that works.
- Database selection needs careful consideration; this will include database availability as many require a subscriptions.
- The search strategy should fit the review question and eligibility criteria.
- Sensitivity and specificity need to be balanced. The first will find a large number of papers but may include many that are irrelevant. The latter will find fewer but has a greater risk of missing papers.
- It is important to understand the database that is being used. This includes how it manages index terms, for example, MeSH terms in MEDLINE/PubMed, and any special characters such as truncation or wildcards.
- The impact of any limits that are applied must be recognised. If in any doubt, repeat the search with and without limits to assess their impact.
- All search strategies should be replicable.

The process of searching the literature is a deceptively complex one. The novice, having been used to searching Google for items of interest, might assume that searching the professional literature is as easy and intuitive—sadly this is not the case. In deciding to undertake a systematic search, you are launching into a sea of different possible search terms, database coverage issues and your own views on the subject that may differ from those of other people. No search strategy will be perfect, and the reviewer may never be fully satisfied. It is easier to show that a search is flawed—one missed paper will confirm that.

Although there is no single right way of doing a search, there are certainly things that can be done wrong. Searching is often an iterative exercise, which means that it usually takes more than one attempt to get it right, and two people searching exactly the same topic will usually construct different searches. As ever, the issue is not whether the reader agrees with the search, but is it well thought out and is it transparent?

© The Editor(s) (if applicable) and The Author(s), under exclusive license to Springer Nature Switzerland AG 2020
E. Purssell, N. McCrae, *How to Perform a Systematic Literature Review*,
https://doi.org/10.1007/978-3-030-49672-2_4

Throughout this book, we have emphasized the importance of methodological consistency and rigour. An exemplar is the Joanna Briggs Institute method [1], which entails a three-stage approach:

1. Identifying the initial keywords to be searched and then looking at these early papers to look for other terms that they have used that might be useful. You might think about this as a scoping search. These are searches that map the existing literature or evidence base, including identifying any gaps or uncertainties, and key definitions [2].
2. Apply this to each database in term, bearing in mind that they may have different terms and syntax.
3. Undertake a hand-search of reference lists of all studies retrieved to look for studies that may be relevant but were not found in the search.

4.1   An Initial Foray

A major consideration in systematic searching is balancing the principles of sensitivity and specificity. A search that is sensitive will be as comprehensive as possible and so find any potentially eligible papers. However, this will probably also reap lots of irrelevant papers. A search that is more specific will be targeted in a way that it identifies only relevant papers, but at the risk of missing some. To illustrate, imagine that you were interested in the treatment of asthma in children. Searching just 'asthma' would be very sensitive and find you every paper about asthma in children, but it would also get you papers about asthma in adults. By contrast, you could try to be more specific by searching 'asthma' and 'children', but this may miss papers about asthma in adolescents.

The previous chapter showed how to pose a review question. The viability of this question and ensuing search strategy may be tentatively tested by use of a research database. A common and readily accessible facility for this is Google Scholar. This website is a collection of articles deemed academic, including not only journal papers but also conference abstracts, technical reports, dissertations and theses. Either the full text or abstract must be freely available. Your search result will be shown in order, as stated by the website: 'Google Scholar aims to rank documents the way researchers do, weighing the full text of each document, where it was published, who it was written by, as well as how often and how recently it has been cited in other scholarly literature' (scholar.google.co.uk/intl/en/scholar/about.html). Papers with the most citations tend to be ranked highest, and this means that recent studies may not appear on the first page of search results. If you want to limit to research published in the past 2 or 3 years, you can filter by time in Google Scholar.

Using Google Scholar for a preliminary search is simple, and you will get a good idea of the amount of literature that exists on your topic. Informed by this activity, you may revise your research question, making it broader or narrower in scope. You will also begin to see what search terms work, informing your strategy for a formal literature search.

Another useful preliminary step is to seek previous literature reviews in PubMed (which we will describe in further detail in this chapter). After typing in topical terms in the search box, you can open any relevant paper that appears in the search result and then click on the 'See Reviews' facility on the right side of the screen.

4.2   Facet Analysis

When you have decided on your review question, this needs to be turned into a searchable strategy. Each element of the question (e.g. population, treatment and outcome) is known as a facet. Facet theory was devised in the 1930s by Indian librarian S.R. Ranganathan, who found that existing bibliographic classifications were inadequate for compound topics [3]. A logical approach to the ordering of knowledge, facet analysis disassembles a topic into its essential parts, finding appropriate terms to represent these parts. Facets should not overlap in content, and each should comprise an exhaustive set of terms. Facets do not always need a specific search. A population may not need to be searched if implicit; for example, in reviewing treatment of prostate or cervical cancer, it is unnecessary to search for men or women, respectively.

Facet analysis is a systematic plan for your search, and we will now demonstrate how this is done. Let's use the following review question:

Is ibuprofen better than paracetamol at treating post-operative pain in children?

This is a directional question, as it asks if one drug is better than the other, rather than simply asking which is best. Although the framing of the question may imply that the reviewers think that the answer will be positive, the review will be conducted with an objectively measurable outcome. From a searching perspective, the interventions are clearly specified and readily identifiable. However, these drugs have both generic and brand names, and paracetamol is generically labelled in the USA as acetaminophen; facet analysis requires all names to be searched. A more awkward element of the research question is in the population. How do you define 'children'? Some classifications and database search facilities include people up to age 18; others stop at 16. Do you want a broad age group that includes studies with older boys and girls who have possibly left school? You may want to restrict the age to match the division between child and adult applied in hospital management, although this will vary between (and possibly within) countries. The next problem is on the specificity of post-operative pain. This could be restricted to one symptom or broadened to include any pain.

As well as using a set of text words (whole or truncated) that you have devised, index terms should also be used. A special vocabulary used by bibliographic databases to categorise each paper, index terms enable you to search for papers on a particular topic in a consistent way. The best-known taxonomy of index terms is the Medical Subject Headings (MeSH) of PubMed/MEDLINE, which we will explain in more detail later in this chapter. As a general point, if you use index terms, it is

Table 4.1 Search terms for review of ibuprofen and paracetamol for post-operative pain in children

Population	Intervention	Control	Outcome
Children undergoing surgery	Ibuprofen	Paracetamol	Pain
Children (text word) Children (index term) Surgery (text word) Surgery (index term) Synonyms for children and surgery	Ibuprofen (text word) Ibuprofen (index term) Synonyms for ibuprofen	Paracetamol (text word) Paracetamol (index term) Acetaminophen (text word) Acetaminophen (index term) Synonyms for paracetamol	Pain (text word) Pain (index term) Synonyms for pain

important to check that the database definition matches what you are seeking; for example, the meaning of the MeSH term 'child' might come as a surprise! Using the PICO configuration to create search terms, the review question 'is ibuprofen better than paracetamol at treating post-operative pain in children?' will include the following terms:

Table 4.1 simply contains words with no linkage; we will show how to meaningfully combine search terms later in this chapter.

4.3 Sources

For a systematic review, there is a general expectation that at least three bibliographic databases will be searched. This depends on the topic and the extent of investigation. The Cochrane manual [4] recommends that in reviewing evidence from experimental trials, you start with the Cochrane Central Register of Controlled Trials (CENTRAL), alongside searches in MEDLINE and Embase as the major generic medical databases. These details will differ of course according to your question and the resources that you have.

For most healthcare reviews, an essential source is MEDLINE, a database of around 5200 health science journals, with a biomedical emphasis. Medline is one of the several informational resources run by the National Center for Biotechnology Information (NCBI) in Bethesda, Maryland. Founded by federal statute in 1988, the NCBI is part of the US National Library of Medicine. The NCBI handbook [5] is a useful resource for healthcare researchers. Alongside MEDLINE is PubMed Central, a full-text archive of biomedical and life sciences journal literature. We should be grateful to the American people for providing this tremendous resource free for all.

The other main database for health sciences is Embase, published by Elsevier. Unlike MEDLINE, Embase is not free, so you are likely to rely on an institutional licence to access it through a library or your employer. Embase claims to cover all journals indexed in MEDLINE and an additional 2900 journals that are not (in particular, pharmacology and European journals). As Embase contains all of the records

Table 4.2 Bibliographic databases for literature reviews

Database	Publisher	Content area
MEDLINE/PubMed	National Library of Medicine (USA)	Biomedicine
Embase	Elsevier	Biomedicine
PsycInfo	American Psychological Association	Psychology, psychiatry
Google Scholar	Google	General
ASSIA (Applied Social Science Index and Abstracts)	ProQuest	Social science
SSCI (Social Science Citation Index)	Clarivate	Social science
CINAHL (Cumulative Index to Nursing and Allied Health Literature)	EBSCO	Nursing and allied health literature
AMED (Allied and Complementary Medicine Database)	Health Care Information Service, British Library	Alternative and complementary medicine
OpenGrey	GreyNet	Science, technology, biomedical science, economics, social science and humanities

that are in MEDLINE, if you have access to Embase, you should theoretically be able to search both simultaneously through Embase although this practice is rare.

Other databases that are more specialised include the Cumulative Index to Nursing and Allied Health Literature (CINAHL) and PsycInfo, a database of behavioural sciences and mental health literature. As with Embase, these require a subscription to access them. A summary of the most commonly used databases is shown in Table 4.2.

There is more than one way of accessing most of these databases. Many educational institutes provide the Ovid or EBSCOhost interfaces. Although these do provide very useful tools and if you have access to them you should consider using them, MEDLINE also has an interface that is free, powerful and accessible from anywhere: PubMed.

4.4 Using PubMed

PubMed is a freely available version of MEDLINE. It could be described as 'MEDLINE plus', because it contains not only MEDLINE but also papers published 'ahead of print', papers yet to be indexed in MEDLINE, open-access journals, older publications not in Medline and some medical/academic books. Most of the functionality is directly available through PubMed, although some features can only be used via Ovid MEDLINE, for which you will depend on institutional subscription. Generally, the openly available PubMed has an intuitive interface that will fulfil most search requirements. For those with previous experience of PubMed, you might find the new interface a little stark; that is because it has been optimised for mobile devices. Don't worry though, all of the familiar features are there. If you click on the Advanced link underneath the search box, that will take you to the 'Advanced Search Builder' which should look far more familiar.

A straightforward way of using PubMed is to go to the homepage (ncbi.nlm.nih. gov/pubmed). Then click on the link for 'Advanced Search Builder'. Your search will have three essential components:

1. The term to be searched, which goes in the box on the right (we use the example of 'Fever')

2. The type of search to be done and where this should be done (in this case a MeSH term and as text words in the title and abstract)

3. The Boolean operator used to combine searches (in this example, 'OR')

4.4.1 Index Terms

The terms to be searched will be determined by your review question, but they should be tuned to make full use of PubMed. While PubMed has various ways of searching for terms, the most important ones are text words and MeSH terms. MeSH is a thesaurus used by the National Library of Medicine for indexing, so that when papers are published, they are tagged to make them identifiable by topic or other categories. If you opt to use the MeSH facility, PubMed will map your search words to a MeSH term and will find all papers indexed with that term. MeSH terms are arranged in a hierarchical structure, with broad terms dividing into more specific terms. Indeed, the logo for MeSH is a tree, analogising the index to trunk, branches and leaves.

When we talk about MeSH terms, there are actually a few different types of term:

• *Descriptors* are terms that reflect the content of the paper; these include main headings and publication types. Each descriptor is defined by scope note.
• *Entry terms* are synonyms or terms that are closely related to descriptors, allowing for different methods of identifying citations. These are not MeSH terms themselves but work to access them.
• *Qualifiers* also known as subheadings can be used to group citations which are about a particular aspect of a subject for exactly anatomy and histology, diagnosis and pharmacology. These subheadings will include a publication type and characteristics of the group being studied, such as age or gender if appropriate.

If you are not sure about a MeSH term, you can consult the MeSH Browser (meshb.nlm.nih.gov/search). It is a good practice to look at the MeSH Browser to ensure that the meaning and coverage of the term is what you expect. A MeSH term may differ from your intuitive notion. For example, the MeSH term 'child' refers to 'a person 6–12 years of age'. Exploring this further, the hierarchical nature becomes clear, the MeSH Browser revealing:

• Persons: Persons as individuals - this comprises:-

   – Age groups: Persons classified by age from birth *which contains*

      Adolescent: A person 13–18 years of age
      Child: A person 6–12 years of age
      Child, preschool: A child between the ages of 2 and 5
      Infant: A child between 1 and 23 months of age

Embase has its indexing system Emtree, which has unique terms (including names of drugs) but also understands MeSH terms.

As one of your key tasks as a reviewer is to be able to define your terms, if you are not sure the MeSH term might be a good place to start this, see if there is a MeSH term, and see how your terms are defined there. Go to the MeSH Browser and type in your term. Unless you know the term exists, it is better to search for all fragments rather than exact match as this will find terms that include at least one fragment of the word (or search string) that you type as opposed to looking for exactly what you type in. The definition of hypertension, according to MeSH, for example, is:

Persistently high systemic arterial BLOOD PRESSURE. Based on multiple readings (BLOOD PRESSURE DETERMINATION), hypertension is currently defined as when SYSTOLIC PRESSURE is consistently greater than 140 mm Hg or when DIASTOLIC PRESSURE is consistently 90 mm Hg or more.

Each of the capitalised terms is a link to another MeSH term to help you really understand your subject.

4.4.2 Text Words

Text words that you devise can be used to search papers in various ways. Normally, the best option is to search in titles and abstracts. If you search for words anywhere in papers, you will probably get many more hits, but this could cause unnecessary work as a large number of irrelevant papers is likely to be found. In PubMed, select 'Title/Abstract' and type your text word into the search box, either in the advanced search with 'All Fields' selected or the basic search window. PubMed will use its Automatic Term Mapping process, matching your word with MeSH terms, journal and authors and investigators, as well as doing an 'All Fields' search. This won't work if your term is wrapped in quotation marks, because PubMed will then search on the exact phrase only. As use of quotation marks bypasses the Automatic Text Mapping facility, their use is not recommended for general searching. Some common terms such as 'a' and 'the' are known as 'stopwords' in PubMed and are not searched.

Reviewers should be aware that PubMed uses American English spelling and terminology. To some extent, Automatic Term Mapping understands other styles of English and terminology used outside North America. For example, if you type 'paracetamol' into the search box without a tag or quotation marks, PubMed maps this as follows: 'acetaminophen' (MeSH Terms) or 'acetaminophen' (All Fields) or 'paracetamol' (All Fields). It is important to check the search details box to see exactly how PubMed has interpreted your search term.

4.4.3   Truncation and Wildcards

In many bibliographic databases, search words can be expanded to include various usage and to reduce the need for multiple terms for the same search topic or category. For example, the terms 'psychology', 'psychological' and 'psychologist' may be found simply by the use of the asterisk symbol. 'Psychol*' would find all of these terms, plus any others beginning with that truncated term. Truncation to 'psych*' would draw in terms of different meaning, such as 'psychiatric' and 'psyche', and thus may be unhelpful. For truncation, the asterisk can be used as a wildcard, denoting any letter, symbol or space. For example, 'health*care' would find 'healthcare', 'health care' and 'health-care'. Another operator is adjacency, which allows you to search terms that occur within a given number of words of each other.

Truncation should be used with caution in PubMed because it subverts Automatic Text Mapping, and wildcards within words and adjacency do not work. In other databases, be sure to check the help menu on the use of wildcards, truncation or adjacency, as these may work differently.

4.4.4   Conditioning the Search

Boolean operators are named after George Boole, an English mathematician who explored the rules of logic. In this context, they refer to the logic of relationships between search terms and between sets of search terms. There are three basic Boolean operators, which in PubMed must be typed in capital letters:

- AND—this will include papers that contain *all* of the search terms
- OR—papers that contain *any* of the search terms
- NOT—used to exclude papers

The 'not' operator is rarely used in practice. The Cochrane manual advises against it due to unforeseen consequences. To illustrate its action, if you specify 'not adult' in a search for studies of children, PubMed will exclude papers with data on children and adults.

If you do not specify a Boolean operator, the default in PubMed is 'and'. In our experience, the use of the wrong Boolean operator is one of the main reasons why searches do not work. In particular, like terms should be combined with 'or', and the unwary reviewer who accepts the default setting is likely to miss many relevant papers (unwittingly, the reviewer has searched for papers that include *all* rather than *any* of the specified terms.

4.4.5   Filtering

There are a range of limits and filters that can be applied to make your search more specific, although these should be used with caution. Filters can limit by publication date and language, although as explained in the previous chapter, you need a good rationale for such restrictions. Perhaps the most commonly used Automatic Text Mapping filters are those that restrict to particular types of study. In PubMed, 'Article Types' filters search results by the methodological MeSH term attached to papers. For some reviews, it may be appropriate to use prepared filtering to enhance sensitivity, specificity or a balance of the two. An example of this is the sensitivity- and precision-maximising filter for PubMed published by the Cochrane Collaboration (work.cochrane.org/pubmed):

> #1 randomized controlled trial [pt]
> #2 controlled clinical trial [pt]
> #3 randomized [tiab]
> #4 placebo [tiab]
> #5 clinical trials as topic [mesh: noexp]
> #6 randomly [tiab]
> #7 trial [ti]
> #8 #1 OR #2 OR #3 OR #4 OR #5 OR #6 OR #7
> #9 animals [mh] NOT humans [mh]
> #10 #8 NOT #9

The letters in brackets after the search term refer to the type of search to be done: 'pt' for publication type, 'tiab' for title and abstract, 'mh' for MeSH heading and 'mesh: noexp' for MeSH heading without automatic explosion. If you are using PubMed, there are prespecified filters for you to use if you wish.

4.4.6   Using PubMed

If you last used PubMed a few years ago, returning to it, you will find it looks and works very differently. Firstly, the default screen is very plain, consisting of only a search box into which you type your search terms. For most searches, it is recommended that you:

- Don't use punctuation such as quotation marks
- Don't use Boolean operators
- Don't use tags

This is because PubMed has a system called Automatic Term Mapping which aims to match words to MeSH terms, journals and then authors. Any phrases and the individual terms within them are also searched as free-text terms in All Fields. For example, if you search children pain PubMed translates that into:

("child"[MeSH Terms] OR "child"[All Fields] OR "children"[All Fields]) AND ("pain"[MeSH Terms] OR "pain"[All Fields])

If you want to construct your search yourself, you can go to the Advanced screen to do this. Here, you can also see the History and Search Details, and by clicking on the Details tab, you can then see the details of how PubMed has structured your search.

By default PubMed uses Best Match to order results, which uses a machine learning algorithm to put the most relevant papers at the top of the results. This can be changed to the most recent on the results page.

To export citations to reference management software, you can do so by clicking Save and then change the format to RIS which can then be saved by clicking Create file. This can then be imported into your reference management software. Citations can also be emailed from that menu or saved into a NCBI account. If you are planning to use PubMed seriously, you should register with the National Center for Biotechnology Information (NCBI) to get a free account. There are many other features here apart from the ability to save searches that you can access through registering and then remembering to log in each time you use PubMed.

PubMed also provides you with some very useful tools. One particularly helpful tool is the Similar Articles feature; to find this, get the paper up on PubMed where you will then find the abstract. If you scroll to the bottom, you will find the Similar articles and articles that have cited the paper; you will also find the MeSH terms and Publication types associated with the paper. There are also a range of Filters which can be found on the left of the search page including article type and publication type.

4.5   Running and Recording Your Search

When you are satisfied with your search specifications in PubMed, click the red 'Search' button, and your search will be run. Look on the right side of the screen for the box marked 'Search Details', which shows exactly how the search was done. This should be saved and appended to your review, as it will allow others to replicate your search. Be sure to keep a detailed record of your search and any amendments that you made, as you will need to report this both in the report.

By registering with NCBI, you can save searches in PubMed. Opening a 'My NCBI' account, you will also have access to various customising features for use with PubMed.

In the report of your systematic review, the *Cochrane Handbook* [4] recommends that you include the following detail on the search:

1. List all databases searched
2. Report the dates of when you searched each database
3. Any language or publication status restrictions
4. Any other data sources searched

5. Any researchers or organisations who were contacted as part of the search
6. 'Hand-searching' of reference lists in papers, journals or conference proceedings

In addition, the full search strategy should be provided as an appendix to the main paper, such that a reader could, if they wished, repeat the search. For further guidance on making the most of PubMed search facilities, see papers by Fatehi et al. [6–8] and the help features of this and the other databases.

4.6   Other Data Sources

4.6.1   Google Scholar

In our experience, students are wary of using Google for a formal search. Don't be! While searching in Google may produce lots of irrelevant or substandard material, this is a problem common to other databases such as MEDLINE and Embase. Inclusion of a paper in a bibliographic database is not a guarantee of quality; maximising this is your responsibility as reviewer. We should consider Google Scholar to be a bibliographic database in its own right, but it is rarely included in the automated search; instead, it may be included in a 'hand-search' alongside perusal of reference lists. Google Scholar, as its name suggests, is a database of scholarly articles (from a wide range of sources but mostly journal papers, conference proceedings, technical reports and dissertations), and either the full text of the articles or abstract must be freely available. As there is no language, journal or geographical restriction, Google Scholar has major benefits in finding literature that is unavailable on other databases. The disadvantage is that internet search engine websites are not updated as immediately as are bibliographic databases such as MEDLINE. Although new papers are added several times per week, some material may not appear for weeks or months after publication. Another problem is that searches conducted in Google Scholar are not as replicable as on conventional bibliographic databases, because the indexing and content of sources may change over time.

4.6.2   Grey Literature

Research literature is not always published in the traditional outlet of academic journals. Technical reports, doctoral theses, conference presentations and official documents may not appear in bibliographic databases (although some will be found on Google Scholar). Known as 'grey literature', there are databases specifically to collate these potentially useful items. OpenGrey, for example, describes itself as 'a multidisciplinary European database, covering science, technology, biomedical science, economics, social science and humanities' (opengrey.eu). You may also find unpublished data from clinical trial registries such as the ISRCTN (International Standard Randomised Controlled Trial Number), which now includes data not only from RCTs but also other types of study (isrctn.com). Unpublished study data and reports are also accessible on Web of Science (clarivate.com/products/web-of-science/web-science-form/web-science-core-collection/) and Scopus (scopus.com).

Two important caveats should be issued about grey literature. Firstly, unpublished reports have not passed through the critical filter of peer review, although we should not assume peer review as a guarantee of quality—because it is not. Secondly, inclusion of grey literature inevitably entails quite nuanced judgements about what to include, inevitably detracting from replication. Therefore, it is crucial to describe clearly the sources, search methods and selection of grey literature.

4.6.3   Reference Management

One of the less glamorous tasks in writing a review is that of reference management. Here we are concerned not with the intellectual cut and thrust of applying inclusion criteria to studies, data extraction or synthesis, but the much more mundane but equally important process of storing, manipulating and sharing the references. Managing large numbers of references can be difficult. If you think about searches that may produce hundreds of papers from different databases and the various manipulations that you will need to do to these including finding duplicates, indicating which meet the inclusion criteria and which not, and then producing a reference list, you will understand that a friendly hand along the way might be helpful. This is where reference management software comes in. You will recall that we saved our PubMed search as a .ris file; this can easily be imported into your reference management software usually through FILE and then IMPORT options.

If you are studying at a college or university, you will probably find that your library or information service centre (or whatever they call it where you are!) will 'support' a particular programme. This just means that they will have a subscription and will know how it works, not that you have to use it. Popular programmes include EndNote, RefWorks, Mendeley and our personal favourite Zotero. We like Zotero for a few reasons: firstly, it is free; secondly, it has very good web integration both in terms of extracting data from websites and that you can access it through a stand-alone programme and a browser; and thirdly, it also enables you to have groups which more than one person can access via the internet. These groups can be open so that anyone can see them, or closed and restricted to nominated members only just as you desire. Zotero also has a browser-only based version called ZoteroBib, which is truly reference management software for people who don't like reference management software. It is not going to be enough for your review if your review is of any great complexity, but if you tell your non-review-producing colleagues about it, they will love you. We have produced a Zotero Groups website for this book where we have listed all of the references so you can see what it looks like—just put this into your browser https://www.zotero.org/groups/2460528/systematicreview-book/library. We think that this is good practice in the spirit of openness and transparency, and we will add new references from time to time.

For more complex reviews, Cochrane have produced their own Covidence programme which can be used for a variety of tasks including reference management and screening and which can be integrated with the other Cochrane programmes (https://www.covidence.org/home). We don't consider this any further here, because our focus is on freely available of low-cost tools and Covidence requires a personal or institutional subscription. There is also an R package known as metagear which will do the same thing [9]. These latter tools are a little different to the software management programmes because they are designed for use by teams for multiple screeners, although a Zotero group could also be used for that purpose as well.

One final thought about using an institutionally supported system, if you are going to leave that institution, make sure that at some point you export your references so that you don't lose them as soon as your access to the institutional support ends. Even if you have not used Zotero for your review, this may be the point to start to use if for storage of references if nothing else, as it will always be freely available to you.

4.7   Conclusion

Literature searching is a systematic but also a creative task. Often it is an iterative process, needing more than one attempt to get it right. Searching is a balance of sensitivity and specificity. All decisions should be transparent: your search should be repeatable by another reviewer based on the step-by-step information that you provide. Remember to keep records of each stage of the search, so that you can report accurately, with numbers to display in the flowchart. There will not be a single correct set of search terms to use in a systematic review, but all decisions should be based on scientific rationale, for the sake of validity, transparency and replicability.

References

1. Lockwood C, Porrit K, Munn Z, Rittenmeyer L, Salmond S, Bjerrum M, Loveday H, Carrier J, Stannard D (2020) Chapter 2: Systematic reviews of qualitative evidence. In: Aromataris E, Munn Z (eds). JBI Manual for Evidence Synthesis. JBI. https://synthesismanual.jbi.global. https://doi.org/10.46658/JBIMES-20-03
2. Armstrong R, Hall BJ, Doyle J, Waters E (2011) "Scoping the scope" of a Cochrane review. J Public Health 33:147–150. https://doi.org/10.1093/pubmed/fdr015
3. Spiteri L (1998) A simplified model for facet analysis: Ranganathan 101. Can J Libr Inform Sci 23:1–30
4. Lefebvre C, Glanville J, Briscoe S, Littlewood A, Marshall C, Metzendorf M-I, Noel-Storr A, Rader T, Shokraneh F, Thomas J, Wieland LS (2019) Chapter 4: Searching for and selecting studies. In: Higgins JPT, Thomas J, Chandler J, Cumpston M, Li T, Page MJ, Welch VA (eds). Cochrane Handbook for Systematic Reviews of Interventions version 6.0 (updated July 2019), Cochrane. https://www.training.cochrane.org/handbook
5. National Center for Biotechnology Information (US) (2013) The NCBI handbook, 2nd edn. National Center for Biotechnology Information (US), Bethesda, MD

6. Fatehi F, Gray LC, Wootton R (2013) How to improve your PubMed/MEDLINE searches: 1. Background and basic searching. J Telemed Telecare 19:479–486. https://doi.org/10.1177/1357633X13512061
7. Fatehi F, Gray LC, Wootton R (2014) How to improve your PubMed/MEDLINE searches: 2. Display settings, complex search queries and topic searching. J Telemed Telecare 20:44–55. https://doi.org/10.1177/1357633X13517067
8. Fatehi F, Gray LC, Wootton R (2014) How to improve your PubMed/MEDLINE searches: 3. Advanced searching, MeSH and My NCBI. J Telemed Telecare 20:102–112. https://doi.org/10.1177/1357633X13519036
9. Lajeunesse MJ (2016) Facilitating systematic reviews, data extraction and meta-analysis with the METAGEAR package for R. Methods Ecol Evol 7:323–330. https://doi.org/10.1111/2041-210X.12472

Screening Search Results: A 1-2-3 Approach

5

Summary Learning Points
- The screening process removes papers that are irrelevant or not required for your review. If the search is not very specific or if it is a popular subject area, there may be a large number of papers.
- This process should normally be undertaken by at least two people working independently to reduce the risk of missing papers or bias in the selection process.
- Papers must be selected on the basis of the question and eligibility criteria.
- A Preferred Reporting Items for Systematic Reviews and Meta-Analyses (or PRISMA) flowchart is a necessity.
- Meticulous record-keeping of numbers and decisions made is important for future reference and replicability.

The bleary-eyed PhD student arrives for a supervision session. The supervisor asks how the literature review is going. The student has had little sleep, having worked into the early hours of the morning sifting through 3000 papers from the database search, eventually finding 25 papers eligible for the review. Then the supervisor finds that a common symptom or treatment was omitted. So the student must repeat the process!

Screening is probably the most labour-intensive stage of systematic reviewing. With a vast and expanding amount of published literature, a reviewer should be braced for a hefty workload. A narrowly focused review question is no guarantee of a small set of relevant papers from the automated search, partly because of the vagaries of indexing, but also due to inconsistent use of terms around the world of research. Like a hamster on a treadmill, the reviewer gets on a momentum, working for hour after hour sorting the search results into 'yes' and 'no'.

E. Purssell, N. McCrae, *How to Perform a Systematic Literature Review*,
https://doi.org/10.1007/978-3-030-49672-2_5

5.1   Reference Management Software

Since the 1980s, when electronic research databases such as Medline emerged, researchers have created bespoke libraries of literature related to their research interests. Reference management software is used to collate and cite literature. Tools such as *EndNote* are basically databases that store full bibliographic references, and they are useful for systematic reviews because they allow a full set of search results to be imported and managed in tasks such as screening. Use of reference management software for the screening process is recommended by the *Cochrane Handbook for Systematic Reviews* [1]. A survey by Lorenzetti and Ghali [2] found that 80% of a sample of 122 published systematic reviews had used such software (over half of the reviewers used *EndNote*).

Reference management software enables the reviewer to combine papers from multiple databases used for the search. Many of the papers will be duplicates, and these can be eliminated almost entirely by automated means. This is just one advantage of reference management applications in the screening process. Although it is not a requirement to use such a tool, it is clearly advantageous to an Excel spreadsheet, which may be used ubiquitously but is not designed for textual data. Reference management applications allow direct linkage to papers. Another practical benefit is that you can easily change the citation style in the report of your review. Journals differ in referencing, and if your initial submission is rejected and you send it elsewhere, it is an irksome task to amend each reference to suit the second journal. The software can change to any citation style on one click!

Which software to use? Most universities have licences to commercial products such as *EndNote* or *Reference Manager*, which run on computers within the licensed institution. These can also be purchased for domestic computer use. Freely available tools include the *Mendeley* and *Zotero*, which both have desktop and online versions. Web-based use is highly flexible as your data are stored in cyberspace rather than on a particular computer or server, but a disadvantage is dependence on Internet speed and susceptibility to connection problems, which can be frustrating for some researchers working at home.

Here is an illustration of importing search results, using *Zotero*. Taking a set of papers found in PubMed, click on 'Send to' and then in 'Choose destination', select 'Citation manager'. This will allow you to save the search result on your computer as a .nbib file, which can be imported into *Zotero* through 'File' and 'Import'. If you have a small number of papers, you could add them manually using the 'Add items by identifier' button (which looks like a wand). Clicking on this will open a box into which you can insert the PubMed identification number (e.g. PMID: 29454216). This will automatically add the citation. You may also use the digital object identifier (DOI) number, which follows the document wherever it is transported. *Zotero* can also identify references by ISBN or ISSN international library numbers.

5.2   Three Stages of Screening

A typical search output would be several thousand items. That's a lot of papers to read! Thankfully you do not need to do this, because a large proportion of the papers will be obviously irrelevant, and these can be excluded simply by viewing the titles. This is the first stage of screening, and it will usually remove more than half of the papers. The second stage is to view the abstracts. Again, this will remove many if not most of the remaining papers. You may rely on the detail of your eligibility criteria to make decisions (e.g. wrong age range). For the final stage, it is necessary to get the full papers. You are not expected to examine every line of text, though. For eligibility, the key section is the method, which will show whether the study is of the relevant population, exposure/intervention and outcome measurement. Rarely, the results section may be needed to confirm eligibility.

5.3   Screening Form

Normally this is a practical procedure whereby reviewers assess papers for inclusion or exclusion. Eligibility requirements may be arranged in the same order as in the research question or PICO formulation. Every box must be ticked for the paper to qualify. This could take the form of a table comprising all of the studies or a sheet to be used for each study. Ultimately, all screening decisions should be collated in one data file. How you do this is your choice; but a record of the whole screening process may be submitted to a journal as a supplementary data file.

If a paper has been found ineligible on a particular criterion, it is not necessary to continue screening on the other eligibility criteria. Consequently, screening data may not be comprehensive but simply show the point at which papers were excluded. Like horses falling at a fence at the Grand National race, typically there will be more casualties at the earlier tests (more failures on population sampling than on outcome measurement).

Reviewers should always err on the side of caution, keeping papers for the next stage of screening if unsure. Therefore, as well as 'yes' and 'no', there should be a 'maybe' category too.

5.4   Sharing the Load

The screening process may be conducted by two or more reviewers, perhaps as a team effort in a funded project. *Zotero* and *Mendeley* enable groups to work together remotely, with live updating of the data. In *Zotero*, web-based entries are synchronised with any number of users' desktop version. Duplicates from the database searches can mostly be remove automatically, although not completely due to differences in indexing of papers.

Covidence [3] is a tool produced by the Cochrane Community to enhance efficiency of screening and other activities in systematic reviews, particularly for large projects involving a team of reviewers. It is free for authors of Cochrane reviews; otherwise an annual fee applies (although a free trial is available). Search results are uploaded to *Covidence* and duplicates are automatically removed. Reviewers on different sites can work individually on the screening process, for example, five reviewers each allocated a fifth of the papers. Screeners can use the annotation facility on the decision dashboard to explain their verdict or inform team discussion. For anyone familiar with the *R* statistical programme, there is a package called *metagear* [4] that can randomly assign papers to screeners, and rate inter-reviewer reliability.

Formal analysis of reliability of screening verdicts by reviewers is not required, although it may add to the rigour of a systematic review. At the very least, papers of uncertain eligibility should be discussed with the chief reviewer for a final decision. It is good practice for a sample of papers screened by each reviewer to be checked by another reviewer. Often there will be discrepancies. Any disagreement should be seen as constructive, as it can help to bolster the eligibility criteria.

5.5   Flowchart

An essential item in reporting a systematic review is a diagrammatic display of the screening process. The PRISMA Statement [5] requires a transparent report of all input and output, from the initial mass of automated search results to the final set of eligible studies for the review. In the standard PRISMA flowchart, all study reports are positioned at the top. It is not a requirement to show the number of papers from each database, but it enhances the information displayed. The next level down shows that the number of papers from automated search after duplicates is removed. Then the three-stage process of screening (by title, by abstract, by full paper) is shown, with a box to the side showing the number of papers discarded. The last box shows the number of papers included in the review. Any additional sources (e.g. studies found in reference lists) are shown as input next to the database totals at the top of the flowchart and added to the final tally.

For demonstration, here is the screening process of a systematic review conducted by one of our PhD students. This was a review of the mental health impact of Internet-based social media use in adolescence. Specifically, the reviewer sought studies that measured both the independent variable (amount of social media use) and dependent variable (depression, anxiety and psychological distress), in general population samples of age 13–18.

The results from automated searches in Medline, Embase, PsycINFO, CINAHL and Social Sciences Citation Index were loaded on a Mendeley reference management file (Fig. 5.1).

You will see that screening reduced the number of papers from thousands to a mere 16. Although there has been an explosion in research on the social and psychological impact of the Internet, the reviewer's strict criteria resulted in merely a third of 1% of the database finds being included. Here are some examples of the excluded papers:

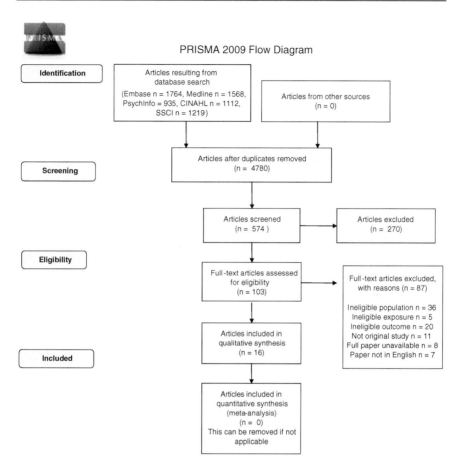

SSCI = Social Sciences Citation Index

Fig. 5.1 Flowchart of screening for review of social media and mental health problems.
SSCI social sciences citation index. (From Moher D, Liberati A, Tetzlaff J, Altman DG, The PRISMA Group (2009) *Preferred Reporting Items for Systematic Reviews and Meta-Analyses*: The PRISMA Statement. PLoS Med 6(7): e1000097. https://doi.org/10.1371/journal. pmed.1000097; www.prisma-statement.org)

- 'A double-edged sword? Psychological distress and internet use in schoolchildren'
  - This was a commentary, not a study.
- 'Online social interaction and mental well-being in adolescents'
  - The title of this study warranted inclusion to the next stage of screening. On reading the abstract, it was confirmed that the outcome variable was too broad (well-being rather than mental health).
- 'Social networking and depression in the young: a cohort study of schoolchildren'

- This study passed screening by title, but the abstract revealed that the age range started too young (11–16). The paper was retained for full text screening, which showed that analysis of the age group required by the reviewer was not separable from that of younger children.
- 'Depressed young people and dependence on Facebook'
  - This study was too selective: participants were chosen on a mental health status that was already known. The sample was not representative. However, studies should not exclude people with existing mental health problems if they are not recruited on that basis.
- 'Social networking sites and depression in an adolescent cohort'
  - This study appeared to fit the review question. However, reading of the method section of the paper showed that participants were chosen on whether they used social media, which was not quantified.

The PhD student was surprised to complete the screening process with so few papers, as this is a topic that has attracted a vast research interest. However, by adhering to the specificity of the review question, the student ended with a set of papers that could be more intensively analysed. More is less!

5.6   Reporting the Screening Outcome

The reviewer should present a summary of the eligible studies. A table providing details of authors, title, study design and results is often placed immediately after the flowchart, within the 'method' section. In principle, this should be reserved for the beginning of the 'results' section (just as a table describing participants should be at the start of a 'results' section in a study report). After confirming eligibility through screening, any scrutiny of the included papers is part of the reviewing process. Everything covered in this and the preceding two chapters was preparation, but now we shall move on to the primary purpose of reviewing the literature.

References

1. Lefebvre C, Glanville J, Briscoe S, Littlewood A, Marshall C, Metzendorf M-I, Noel-Storr A, Rader T, Shokraneh F, Thomas J, Wieland LS (2019) Chapter 4: Searching for and selecting studies. In: Higgins JPT, Thomas J, Chandler J, Cumpston M, Li T, Page MJ, Welch VA (eds). Cochrane Handbook for Systematic Reviews of Interventions version 6.0 (updated July 2019), Cochrane. https://www.training.cochrane.org/handbook
2. Lorenzetti DL, Ghali WA (2013) Reference management software for systematic reviews and meta-analyses: an exploration of usage and usability. BMC Med Res Methodol 13:141. https://doi.org/10.1186/1471-2288-13-141
3. Cochrane Community Covidence. https://community.cochrane.org/help/tools-and-software/covidence. Accessed 17 Apr 2020
4. Lajeunesse MJ (2016) Facilitating systematic reviews, data extraction and meta-analysis with the metagear package for R. Methods Ecol Evol 7:323–330. https://doi.org/10.1111/2041-210X.12472
5. Moher D, Liberati A, Tetzlaff J et al (2009) Preferred reporting items for systematic reviews and meta-analyses: the PRISMA statement. PLoS Med 6:e1000097. https://doi.org/10.1371/journal.pmed.1000097

Critical Appraisal: Assessing the Quality of Studies

6

Summary Learning Points
- Critical appraisal of papers is important, as it allows readers to understand the strengths and limitations of the literature.
- The first thing that should be considered is the quality of reporting of individual studies; do they provide sufficient information?
- The quality of the method and conduct of the individual studies is concerned with methodological quality.
- Within the broad consideration of quality, there is the specific concept of risk of bias which should be explicitly considered.
- Critical appraisal is a little different in qualitative research, but the principles still apply.
- Various tools exist, some of which are specific to types of review question such as Cochrane or Joanna Briggs Institute, while others are not.

6.1 Assessing Quality

You may have an idea of what 'quality' means in your daily life. Is an item of clothing to your taste, well made, and is it reasonably priced? Was the film you saw at the cinema worth watching? The idea of quality when the product is primary research or indeed a systematic review is harder to define, however. Scientific standards should apply, yet there is no single dimension of quality in research; rather there are four related but distinct types of quality, which may be assessed at two levels. We refer to 'two levels' because there are separate assessments of each individual study and all of the studies together, just as there are medals for different events at the Olympics and an overall medal table for each country. In this analogy the individual events are the studies, and each country represents a body of evidence in the review.

E. Purssell, N. McCrae, *How to Perform a Systematic Literature Review*,
https://doi.org/10.1007/978-3-030-49672-2_6

1. Quality of reporting—of individual studies and of the review
2. Quality of the method and conduct—of individual studies and of the review
3. Risk of bias—in individual studies and in the review
4. Quality of the body of evidence

It is important to look at these two levels separately because, to put it bluntly, you can do a bad job of doing a review of good papers or more positively a good one with poorer papers. In this chapter, we shall focus on the critical appraisal of the individual studies, which is a crucial stage before going on to analyse the study findings. We will discuss issues surrounding the appraisal of the body of evidence in Chap. 9.

6.2   Critical Appraisal

At the outset we should make an important differentiation between critical appraisal and criticism. Critical appraisal is the balanced assessment of a piece of research, looking for its strengths and weaknesses and then coming to a balanced judgement about its trustworthiness and its suitability for use in a particular context. If this all seems a bit abstract, think of an essay that you submit to pass a course. The process of marking is to look at the good and not so good aspects of your essay and to come to an overall judgement about them, for example, is it factually correct and clearly written (this is the trustworthiness part), but then to see if you have answered the actual question (this is the contextual part). Critical appraisal, like marking essays, is a systematic and balanced process, not one of simply looking for things to criticise.

6.3   Hierarchies of Evidence

You might intuitively think that some types of study or evidence are 'better' than others, and it is true that certain of evidence are evidentially stronger than others. Just as an eyewitness is 'better' than circumstantial evidence. However, there is an important qualification here, which is what you are looking for is not necessarily a theoretical generic 'ideal study' but the best type of study that could be done to answer your question. This idea of some types of evidence being better is reflected in what are known as 'hierarchies of evidence' which you can think of as being like a league table of evidence types. There are many such hierarchies that have been published, for example, that by the Oxford Centre for Evidence-Based Medicine [1].

For quantitative research a typical hierarchy might be:

1. *Systematic review of randomised controlled trials*—systematic reviews are always a higher level of evidence than an individual study because they look at all of the literature on a subject in a systematic manner. They should be done using a recognised methodology and be transparent so you know not just what the authors have done but also why they have done it. So a systematic review of

randomised controlled trials (RCT) is a higher level than an individual RCT, a systematic review of cohort studies is a higher level of evidence than an individual cohort study and so on.

2. *Randomised controlled trials*—the three defining features of an RCT, namely, randomisation between interventions, having a control group, and manipulation of a variable make these the strongest level of individual study evidence. Really we should differentiate between what we might refer to as a random sample-random allocation controlled trial (RRCT) from RCT not having a random sample, as random sampling is also very important for reasons we will discuss in Chap. 7. However, as the conduct of interventions used in an RCT is not always the same as the context in which they are used in clinical practice, they often show efficacy (answering the question 'can it work?') rather than effectiveness ('does it work in practice?'). Many questions also cannot be answered using these types of study for practical or ethical reasons as randomisation is not possible.

3. *Nonrandomised controlled trials*—because these lack randomisation between intervention groups, there is an increased risk of bias making them a lower level of evidence than an RCT.

4. *Systematic reviews of prospective observational studies*—these are here for the same reason that a systematic review of RCT evidence was at the first level.

5. *Prospective observational studies*—because interventions are not manipulated and the participants are not randomised between groups, these studies have a higher risk of bias and so are lower in the hierarchy. However, many questions can only be answered using observational studies making these the best type of study for such questions. If you are going to do an observational study, prospective data collection, where you collect data as you go, is better than retrospective data use because it means you can plan data collection and ensure that it is accurately collected and managed. You may hear these referred to as prospective cohort studies.

6. *Systematic review of retrospective observational studies.*

7. *Retrospective observational studies*—these are similar to the observational studies referred to in level 5, but the data is used retrospectively. Because you are relying on data that has already been collected and often for quite different purposes, you may find that the data are not complete or accurate. Case-control studies are found at this level, along with retrospective cohort studies.

8. *Case reports/case series*—these are single or multiple reports about something of interest and usually do not have any kind of comparison group. These are often the very earliest reports of new phenomena and can be used to generate hypotheses but not to test them.

9. *Expert opinion*—this is not really a level of evidence but an interpretation of evidence; experts are experts because they know things or have had particular experiences. The important thing here is to establish on what this opinion is based, is it based on experience, research or something else? Be clear; this is not to decry or diminish expert opinion but just that it should be seen for what it is. Expert opinion is very important, and one very important use of this is the opinion of patients, carers and others receiving the interventions that we are reviewing.

Ordering qualitative research designs by quality is debatable due to the differing philosophical and epistemological rationale [2]. However it may be helpful to have some idea of the equivalent of this hierarchy for qualitative research [3], although the levels here are identified at a more general level rather than identifying specific methods:

1. *Generalisable studies*—these studies are characterised by having a sampling strategy clearly focussed and informed by a comprehensive literature review, sampling being extended if necessary to capture the full diversity of the phenomena under investigation. The analysis is clear and comprehensive, although this may be in supplementary information if journal word count does not allow full explanation. The relevance of the findings to other settings are made and clearly discussed.
2. *Conceptual studies*—these studies base sampling on clear theoretical concepts, but the sample may not as diverse as level 1 studies. The analysis comprises an account of the views of the participants, with appropriate conclusions drawn from these. Diversity in views is recognised but is limited to one group or a number of subgroups, and data saturation may not be achieved.
3. *Descriptive studies*—these studies tend not to be based on theory but are usually descriptive and look at views or experiences in a specific group or setting. As a consequence of this, there is no further sampling diversity, and so the ability to generalise findings is very limited.
4. *Single case study*—these studies provide data on only one subject and so cannot be generalised to others. They may however be useful in developing hypotheses.

Let us now consider the three broad aspects of quality (reporting, methodological and risk of bias) in more detail.

6.4   Quality of Reporting

The first of these types of quality is to do with how well the study is reported. Reporting guidelines are important tools for authors, editors and reviewers. They have been defined as 'a checklist, flow diagram, or structured text to guide authors in reporting a specific type of research, developed using explicit methodology' [4]. That is to say they tell you what should be in a paper and give you some idea of the order in which these things should be presented. Although they vary quite widely in their format, what they have in common is that they will have been developed using an explicit methodology, that is to say, you know who developed them and how they were developed. You would also hope that they have been tested in some way, although many are really only based on consensus.

There are now a very large number of these reporting guidelines for different methodologies and different subtypes of methodologies in some cases. There are so many now that they now need their own website, which is known as the EQUATOR (Enhancing the QUAlity and Transparency Of health Research) Network. The most common reporting guidelines for individual studies that you are likely to come across are: CONSORT (Consolidated Standards of Reporting Trials) for randomised studies [5]; STROBE (Strengthening the Reporting of Observational Studies in Epidemiology) for observational studies [6]; and AGREE II (Appraisal of Guidelines for RE and Evaluation II) for guidelines [7]. For your review the reporting guidance for each individual study is probably not so important unless there is insufficient information in the paper for you to use it, in which case you should probably not use it anyway. They are really most used by authors who want to make sure that they have included everything and journal editors and reviewers who also want to check this. If you think that there is something missing from a paper, you may find them useful to check if this is important, and some journals now publish the completed checklists with papers as supplementary files. What you must do is to resist the temptation to use reporting guidance as a quality appraisal tool—they were not designed for this purpose.

The one set of reporting guidelines that you will definitely want to know about is that for systematic reviews, because you will need this when you write up and submit yours, whether this is to a journal or as an assignment. The reporting guidelines for systematic reviews are known as PRISMA, which stands for the **P**referred **R**eporting Items for **S**ystematic Reviews and **M**eta-**A**nalyses [8]. The full package includes the PRISMA flowchart which you will have seen if you have read a systematic review, a checklist and the full paper explaining the tool and how to use it. When you submit your review, either for publication or for marking, you should complete the PRISMA flowchart and checklist. These should either be submitted in the text of the document, or as an appendix depending upon the requirements of the journal or course. We will return to PRISMA in Chap. 10.

One important point to bear in mind is the differing requirements of journals, and if you are ever not sure about how a paper is presented, look for the instructions for authors for that journal. This will be found somewhere on the journal website, and it should explain why things are set out in the way that they are. Some journals are very prescriptive about what can and cannot go in the paper, so if you think there is something missing, always check these instructions. The most common thing that is missing is probably confirmation of ethical approval; this is nearly always confirmed at the point of submission, and so it may be thought to be a waste of valuable journal space if there are no particular issues that require discussion. There may also be supplementary information where important information may be found.

6.5   Methodological Quality of Studies

The assessment of a studies methodological quality is looking at how well the study has been designed and conducted. Remember that here we are just concerned with the individual studies. You may be more used to the term 'critical appraisal', and if so that is fine; it is much the same thing. There is a difference in how this is assessed in the two systematic review methodologies produced by the Cochrane Collaboration and the Joanna Briggs Institute (JBI). While the Cochrane process concentrates on risk of bias and clearly differentiates this from wider concepts of quality or critical appraisal [9], the JBI combines critical appraisal and assessment of risk of bias stating that the purpose of this 'is to assess the methodological quality of a study and to determine the extent to which a study has excluded or minimized the possibility of bias in its design, conduct and analysis' [2]. We will return to assessment of the risk of bias in the next section, but what this is probably really showing is the different background to the methodological approaches, Cochrane having its roots in quantitative research and JBI being more focussed on qualitative and mixed methods.

There are a variety of different methodological critical appraisal tools, including those provided by the JBI and another organisation known as the Critical Appraisal Skills Programme (CASP) [2, 10]. Cochrane is not really concerned with broader concept of quality, and so doesn't provide general critical appraisal tools. These tools are methodology specific; this is important because what marks a methodologically sound RCT is different to that for an observational study and different again to a qualitative study. You may see some tools that aim to help you to assess a variety of different study types; you should really avoid these because of this methodological specificity, sometimes in seeking to cover everything a bit you end up covering nothing very comprehensively. As an example, the CASP tool for qualitative studies is shown below (Table 6.1).

One of the problems with all of these critical appraisal tools is that users are not always clear as to what they are actually assessing; sometimes they are assessing bias, other times imprecision, relevance, applicability, ethics and completeness of reporting [9]. These are distinct concepts with different meanings and implications, and they are sometimes important at different times in the review process. For example, the Joanna Briggs Institute Qualitative Critical Appraisal Tool contains the item: 'Is the research ethical according to current criteria or, for recent studies, and is there evidence of ethical approval

Table 6.1 The CASP checklist for qualitative research

Section A: Are the results valid?
1. Was there a clear statement of the aims of the research?
2. Is a qualitative methodology appropriate?
Is it worth continuing?
3. Was the research design appropriate to address the aims of the research?
4. Was the recruitment strategy appropriate to the aims of the research?
5. Was the data collected in a way that addressed the research issue?
6. Has the relationship between researcher and participants been adequately considered?
Section B: What are the results?
7. Have ethical issues been taken into consideration?
8. Was the data analysis sufficiently rigorous?
9. Is there a clear statement of findings?
Section C: Will the results help locally?
10. How valuable is the research?

by an appropriate body?' which is important, but not necessarily a marker of quality in the context of the really important question of whether the results are likely to be right.

It can also be difficult to know how to summarise the results of a critical appraisal; summary scores where you give each study a score of 1 for a requirement being met and 0 if it not met is problematic for two reasons. Firstly each item of a checklist such as those from CASP has different implications for the study and any conclusions that you draw which cannot be seen in a simple numeric score. Secondly some of the items are more important than others and so would need some kind of weighting in the summary score which would be theoretically and practically difficult. For reporting purposes we suggest a table where each study is in a row and each column a different criterion from the checklist. The resulting study-criterion cell in the table can then be coloured green for 'yes' (or the positive response if different), red for 'no' and yellow for 'unclear/don't know'. The size of the treatment effect and precison can be similarly graded with green indicating a large effect and precise estimate. An example of this is shown in Fig. 6.1.

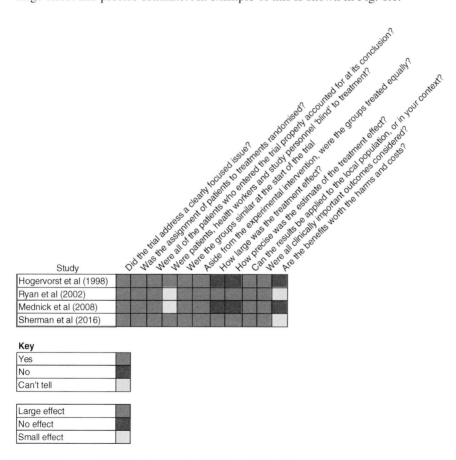

Fig. 6.1 An example of how to present critical appraisal results

6.6   Risk of Bias

For quantitative studies this is the most important part of the appraisal process. Bias in general terms can be defined as 'systematic error, or deviation from the truth, in results' [11] and again can occur at two levels, bias in the results of the individual studies and bias in the results of your review. You may also hear it referred to as internal validity, just be clear to differentiate this from external validity, which is the generalisability of the results to situations that are different from those of the research. As a reviewer biases in the individual studies are beyond your control, although there are ways to mitigate this through transparently reporting the risk of bias and adjusting your recommendations or conclusions accordingly. However, as well as biases within the studies, there are additional factors that can introduce bias at the level of the review, some of which you *can* do something about. At this point it is important to note the language that we are using here—we refer to *risk* of bias rather than actual bias because we don't usually know its extent, just that there is some level of risk of it [9]. There is a very important lesson here, which is to never claim more than what you actually have evidence for. We are also careful when assessing the risk of bias to really think about the risk of *material* bias; that is to say we are really only worried about factors that are likely to affect the result that we are interested in [11].

Bias must also be differentiated from imprecision. The former is due to systematic error, the latter random error [12]. To understand the importance of this, recall that the purpose of quantitative research is to take data from a sample, and to use that to say something about a population, this is what we call inference. What we would like is for our sample result to be a very precise estimate of that population value. If you were to do 100 studies on the same subject, each randomly selecting 50 participants from the same population, you will, of course, get 100 slightly different results as each time you would get 100 different participants. What you are seeing here is sampling error, and the more you have of it, the less precise your results will be.

Although it is called sampling error, it is not an error in the sense of it being a mistake; it is just the variation that you would get from having different samples with different participants. In fact not only is it not a mistake; it is actually both helpful and predictable for reasons that we will discuss in Chap. 6. The important thing is that the result of a study can largely take this type of error into account through the standard error, confidence interval and associated *p*-value [12]. This variation is not bias because it is the result of random error (just who happens to be in the sample). Bias is systematic error, that is, it is something to do with the conduct of the study itself. With a biased methodology, if you did 100 studies, you would get 100 different *and* wrong results. The random error to which we refer to here does have a name; it is called *imprecision*, and we will refer to it later when we discuss GRADE.

6.7   Choosing a Tool

The tool that you use needs to reflect the methodology of the studies that you are using. One of the key things that the reader of your review will want to know is that you understand the studies you are reading, and using the wrong tool is a giveaway that you *don't* really understand them. In both the CASP and JBI methods, a range of tools are available and are clearly marked.

6.7.1 Study-Level Assessment

For quantitative studies we differentiate randomised from nonrandomised studies. This is because the risk of bias is somewhat different between them. Just to be clear, random allocation between treatments is one of the major protections against bias, and this by definition is missing in nonrandomised studies. As we will see later on, this affects not only the study-level assessment of bias but also the overall assessment of the body of evidence. The two main tools for assessing risk of bias at the study level are the Cochrane Risk of Bias Tool-2 (RoB2) [11, 13] and the Risk Of Bias In Non-randomised Studies of Interventions (ROBINS-I) [14], respectively.

6.7.2 Randomised Studies: Cochrane Risk of Bias Tool-2

The new Cochrane Risk of Bias Tool-2 [11, 13], often referred to as RoB2, has five domains to assess the risk of bias. Doing this allows you to come to a conclusion about the overall risk of bias in the study; these are shown in Table 6.2. For those who are familiar with the original Cochrane tool, you will see some of the names are different; the new names have been designed to be more descriptive of the cause of bias that they seek to assess. Each domain has a number of signalling questions, the answers to which are: yes, probably yes, probably no, no and no information. The answers to these questions then inform the decision for the domain, the judgement of which is low risk of bias, some concerns or high risk of bias. If all of the domains are judged to have a low risk of bias, the overall judgement for the study is that it is at a low risk of bias; if there is some risk of bias in

Table 6.2 RoB2 and ROBINS-I compared

RoB2 domains	ROBINS-I domains	Notes
Bias arising from the randomisation process		Nonrandomised studies do not randomise
	Bias due to confounding	If a study is properly randomised, these will be minimised by this process
	Bias in selection of participants into the study	
	Bias in classification of interventions	
Bias due to deviations from intended interventions	Bias due to deviations from intended interventions	These are similar between randomised and nonrandomised studies
Bias due to missing outcome data	Bias due to missing data	
Bias in measurement of the outcome	Bias in measurement of outcomes	
Bias in selection of the reported result	Bias in selection of the reported result	

any domains but not enough to cause serious concern, the judgement would be some concerns; while if a study has a high risk of bias in at least one domain or it has some concerns for multiple domains in a way that causes you to think there may be bias, the judgement would be that there is a high risk of bias. As an option you can also include the predicted direction of bias, is it likely to favour the intervention or the control treatment? There are different questions for randomised parallel-group trials, cluster-randomised parallel-group trials (including stepped-wedge designs) and randomised cross-over trials and other matched designs. For cluster-randomised trials, there is an additional domain, which is *bias arising from identification or recruitment of individual participants within clusters.*

6.7.3 ROBINS-I

For nonrandomised studies of interventions (NRSI), the situation is somewhat different because by definition one of the major protections against bias, that of random allocation between interventions, is missing. To assess risk of bias in these studies, one could use ROBINS-I. This approach sees nonrandom studies as attempting to mimic or emulate a 'hypothetical pragmatic randomised trial, conducted on the same participant group and without features putting it at risk of bias, whose results would answer the question addressed by the NRSI', and so bias in this context is 'a systematic difference between the results of the NRSI and the results expected from the target trial' [14, p. 2]. Importantly this target trial does not have to be ethical or feasible; it is just used as a comparator.

This tool has seven domains, the first three of which are different from RoB2 because these are the domains that deal with issues around the lack of randomisation which are clearly not applicable to RCTs. The remaining four domains are largely the same to RoB2 as the issues are largely the same. These are shown in Table 6.2. Again there are signalling question with the following possible answers: yes, probably yes, probably no, no and no information. For the domain and study-level decisions, the options are low risk of bias (the study is comparable to a well-performed randomised trial); moderate risk of bias (the study provides sound evidence for a nonrandomised study but cannot be considered comparable to a well-performed randomised trial); serious risk of bias (the study has some important problems); critical risk of bias (the study is too problematic to provide any useful evidence and should not be included in any synthesis); and no information on which to base a judgement about risk of bias.

ROBINS-I is relatively new. You may be more familiar with the Newcastle-Ottawa Scale, which is widely used for cohort and case-control studies [15] and is shown in Table 6.3, while RoB2 is replacing the existing Cochrane Risk of Bias Tool. You can see RoB2 and ROBINS-I compared in Table 6.2. It is fair to say that the new tools are more complicated than the older ones and will take more time to complete. Whether you use these new tools or not is probably going to be based on the methodology that you use and the requirements of your course or target journal.

Table 6.3 Newcastle-Ottawa Scales for cohort and case-control studies

Cohort studies	Case-control studies
Selection	
Representativeness of the exposed cohort	Is the case definition adequate?
Selection of the nonexposed cohort	Representativeness of the cases
Ascertainment of exposure	Selection of controls
Demonstration that outcome of interest was not present at start of study	Definition of controls
Comparability	
Comparability of cohorts on the basis of the design or analysis	Comparability of cases and controls on the basis of the design or analysis
Exposure	
Assessment of outcome	Ascertainment of exposure
Was follow-up long enough for outcomes to occur	Same method of ascertainment for cases and controls
Adequacy of follow-up of cohorts	Non-response rate

6.8 Reliability and Validity

There are two key concepts underlying most of what we have just looked at, which are reliability and validity. As with the term quality, you probably have an idea of what these mean in your everyday life, but take care as they have specific meanings in research. Saying Niall is a reliable co-author is using the term reliable is a different way to the one used in research, for example.

6.8.1 Reliability

This is defined as the degree to which results obtained by a particular measurement technique can be replicated [16]. Unlike bias which is to do with systematic error, reliability is a matter of random error. Examples of this might be two people looking at a paper and thinking it has different results, a nurse taking a temperature twice on the same person and getting different results or a set of scales that seems to weight a bit differently every time you use them. The biggest issue of reliability in a systematic review is probably that of random error or variation in selecting papers and data extraction. For example, two people looking at the same table and one person mistaking a 5 for a 6. This is not the same as getting the search wrong in the first place, for example, by using the term hyperthermia in place of fever (they are different!). That would be a systematic error as it will affect all of the papers, and so is an issue of bias.

6.8.2 Validity

Validity is remarkably complex, despite the apparently straightforward definitions you will find in textbooks. Often validity is defined as the extent to which the study really measures what it was intended to measure. This is an oversimplification because validity is much more than that; it is actually the degree to which evidence and theory support the adequacy and appropriateness of the interpretations and actions that come from the results or test scores [17]. That is to say that validity is not really a property of a tool or scale but of the way that a tool or scale is used and the inferences and subsequent actions that come from its use. We often hear students speaking of a 'validated tool', when they are using the tool in a very different way and making very different inferences from those intended by the original authors.

Deconstructing this term a little, we can see that there are two main aspects to validity, these being internal and external validity. We have already met internal validity under a different guise, as it is the degree to which a result is free from bias [11], and it is the assessment of this that tools such as the RoB2, ROBINS-I and Newcastle-Ottawa Scale are concerned with. The second type of validity, often referred to as external validity or generalisability, is the degree to which you can take data from a given sample and apply it in different settings. This is crucial if you are going to bring together different studies in a systematic review because this assumes studies are generalisable enough for them to be combined in this way. To understand this idea of external validity in more detail, you might like to look at Chap. 6 which begins with a discussion of inferential statistics and goes on to consider *heterogeneity* where studies may not be sufficiently generalisable to be combined in a review.

6.9   Qualitative Studies

So far we have focussed on quantitative research. Quality appraisal in qualitative research is different in some ways, but the principles are fundamentally the same. Both approaches should answer a research question through scientific reasoning and methodological rigour. In this section we will be taking two broad approaches to qualitative evidence: one that sees quality in qualitative research as being something quite different from that discussed in quantitative research and the other that sees some similarities. Actually it has been suggested that there are four approaches to this [18]:

1. *The replication perspective* which sees validity as a concept that does apply to qualitative research, even if the way it is assessed may be different.
2. *The parallel perspective* which says that qualitative research really needs different criteria to assess this.
3. *The diversification of meanings perspective* which suggests different approaches depending upon the specific context of studies.
4. *The letting go perspective* which seeks to abandon validity as a concept for qualitative research and to find other criteria upon which to evaluate studies.

We make no recommendation here but present information to allow you to make your own judgement.

6.9.1   Why Might Reliability and Validity Apply Differently in Qualitative Research?

A qualitative study is a creative endeavour relying heavily on the insights and analytic interpretations of the investigator. If two researchers did the same study, the findings would differ to some extent, although overall conclusions should be similar. Each qualitative study is unique, because its participants, setting and the researcher are unique. This is quite unlike the objectivity and replicability of quantitative research. However, there should be transparency in qualitative studies through careful recording of decisions in design, fieldwork and analysis. This makes the study open to critical appraisal and potentially boosts confidence in the findings. It would probably not be unfair to state that much of the qualitative research in academic journals lacks transparency, as shown by a recent review of management studies [19].

Quality of qualitative research can be assessed using criteria somewhat related to those used in quantitative research. These differences were summarised by Lincoln and Guba [20] in Table 6.4 below.

Here is how you apply naturalistic criteria in assessing qualitative studies [21]:

- *Credibility*—does the representation of data fit the views of the participants? Otherwise it is doubtful whether they are true. For critical appraisal look for sufficiency of verbatim quotes, due attention to contrary cases. Credibility may be enhanced by participant validation, although this is not a requirement in all qualitative studies.
- *Transferability*—as generalisability in qualitative research is contextual, there must be adequate description of the study setting, participants and circumstances so that readers can judge whether the findings are transferable to other settings. Transferability is not dichotomous: some contextual factors may be similar, while others may differ between the study setting and comparable settings elsewhere.
- *Dependability*—the process of research should be clearly documented, both in the design and in decisions made in the conduct of the study. For critical appraisal you should be looking for an audit trail. Some qualitative researchers use inter-rater validation of coding or components of the analysis.

Table 6.4 Trustworthiness of findings: scientific and naturalistic criteria

Criterion	Conventional scientific term	Naturalistic term	Naturalistic definition
Truth	Internal validity	Credibility	Confidence in veracity of data and findings: relates to performance of researcher as instrument
Applicability	External validity	Transferability	Extent to which findings may be generalised to other settings
Consistency	Reliability	Dependability	Stability of findings across data set
Neutrality	Objectivity	Confirmability	Findings not biased by personal beliefs (other researchers would produce similar conclusions from data)

- *Confirmability*—to what extent are the findings verifiable? This can be assessed by the grounding of interpretation and themes in the data and through examination of the audit trail. There should be some account of reflexivity, considering the researcher's influence on the findings (including information on the researcher's background, education and perspective).

6.10   Risk of Bias in Qualitative Research: Dependability and Credibility

For those who do think that validity, in whatever way you choose to define it, has a place within qualitative research, there is a tool within the JBI method that looks at the dependability and credibility of findings—the ConQual tool [22]. This contains five items from the JBI-Qualitative Assessment and Review Instrument critical appraisal tool to assess dependability and then assess three levels of credibility; these are shown in Table 6.5. These are aspects of studies that are equivalent to reliability and internal validity in quantitative research, respectively. Although really designed for findings, rather than each study, this does get around the fact that the JBI critical appraisal tool is not equivalent to any of the risk of bias tools discussed as it contains items with no relevance to bias or its qualitative equivalent and it would appear to deal with equivalent concepts to the risk of bias tools. The authors of the paper proposing this tool note that dependability 'can be established by assessing the studies in the review using the above criteria' [22, p. 4].

Another approach is to base assessment of quality in qualitative research not just on method but rather on the conceptual clarity and interpretive rigour. Conceptual clarity refers to how clearly the author has articulated a concept that facilitates theoretical insight and the interpretive rigour to whether the authors interpretation 'be trusted'. For interpretive rigour there are three further categories to aid judgement, as shown in Table 6.6 [23].

Table 6.5 ConQual—factors affecting dependability and credibility

Factors affecting dependability	Factors affecting credibility
Is there congruity between the research methodology and the research question or objectives?	Unequivocal (findings accompanied by an illustration that is beyond reasonable doubt and therefore not open to challenge)
Is there congruity between the research methodology and the methods used to collect data?	Equivocal (findings accompanied by an illustration lacking clear association with it and therefore open to challenge)
Is there congruity between the research methodology and the representation and analysis of data?	Unsupported (findings are not supported by the data)
Is there a statement locating the researcher culturally or theoretically?	
Is the influence of the researcher on the research, and vice versa, addressed?	

Table 6.6 Factors affecting interpretive rigour

Core facet	Categories for interpretive rigour
Conceptual clarity	
Interpretive rigour	What is the context of the interpretation?
	How inductive is the interpretation?
	Has the researcher challenged their interpretation?

The authors then suggest that papers can then be put into one of four categories:

1. Key paper that is 'conceptually rich and could potentially make an important contribution to the synthesis'
2. Satisfactory paper
3. Fatally flawed
4. Irrelevant to the synthesis

6.11 How to Use Your Appraisal Results

How should your critical appraisal be reported? In order to maintain transparency, you should document your decisions and in particular note anything that may reduce the confidence that you have in the results of the studies and ultimately of your review. We suggest either a table of appraisal findings or that you produce a spreadsheet with studies arranged in rows with columns for each question. The corresponding cells can then be coloured green, yellow or red depending upon the answers to each of the question. This would make the presentation analogous to that used for the Cochrane Risk of Bias Tool. Footnotes can then be added to explain your decisions. Tables are easier, but they can be a bit wordy and hard to follow. Ultimately the point of doing this is to inform your decision-making and to make this clear to the reader. We will see how your critical appraisal supports this in Chap. 9.

6.12 What's Next?

You might ask yourself having presented your assessment what else do you do with the resultant information about the quality of the studies in your review. Although you should present the information, ideally, in tabular form and discuss these results; this is not enough on its own. However, in many cases this is all that is done, and there is little evidence that having done all of this work that many authors actually use the information in the synthesis. Remember that undertaking a review is a process whereby each stage should be informed by those that have gone before, and so in this case your quality assessment should inform the synthesis and conclusions which follow it. The most commonly used methods for incorporating the results of quality assessment into reviews include narrative assessment, sensitivity analysis and restricting the synthesis to those studies which are considered higher quality [24].

6.12.1 Narrative Assessment

This is a very broad term that can mean just about anything but usually means some kind of discussion of quality issues in the text. Doing a narrative assessment still requires some kind of tool to be used, and as with other ill-defined narrative aspects, these assessments are sometimes not clear or transparent. It is important to remember that all quality assessments require a narrative explanation of the process and results.

6.12.2 Sensitivity Analysis

This is another broad term referring to the process of repeating the analysis using different decisions or ranges of values where the original choices were made on criteria that were arbitrary or unclear. These decisions occur at many points in the review process, and you should always consider if your choices are likely to make a material impact upon the results of your analysis. The Cochrane handbook suggests, for example, that the effect of study design could be a matter for which a sensitivity analysis is required [25]. You could look to see the effect of including blinded and unblinded studies, the inclusion of only studies meeting a prespecified risk of bias or any other methodological criteria of interest. It is important to differentiate this process from formal subgroup analysis. Subgroup analysis involves formal statistical comparisons between groups, involving the calculation of effect size estimates for each group; this type of sensitivity analysis does not. It simply asks the question: 'what if?'

Although in many places we have emphasised the importance of the process proceeding according to a prespecified plan or protocol, this is an example where this may not be possible. Some reasons for doing a sensitivity analysis may not become clear until the studies have been retrieved and read. The important thing is that you have a good rationale for doing this, which is that you are looking to see how much your results would be affected had you made different decisions during the review process. If the results are not very different, it suggests that your review is robust to these decisions and your results can be considered to have a higher degree of certainty [26].

6.12.3 Restriction to Higher-Quality Studies

If you have read the section above, you will realise that this is just a form of sensitivity analysis, answering the question: do studies with higher quality give a different result to those with lower quality? remembering all of the issues that we highlighted with regard to the idea of 'quality'.

6.13 Conclusion

If quality assessment appears to be complex, that's because it is! The concept of 'quality' is somewhat nebulous, and it is not consistently assessed in systematic reviews [24]. In a four-step approach, this chapter has focused on assessing quality of design and conduct of studies and the specific consideration of bias. We attend to the overall quality of evidence from the reviewed studies (the fourth stage of quality appraisal) in Chap. 9. We would like to make a plea for this not to become just a 'tick box' exercise but one that really interrogates the papers to find out what they are really saying, or not. For students who find this a bit dull, imagine yourself as a famous detective following the clues to the underlying truth:

> The world is full of obvious things which nobody by any chance observes.
> Arthur Conan Doyle (1902)
> *The Hound of the Baskervilles*

References

1. Oxford Centre for Evidence-Based Medicine (OCEBM) (2016) OCEBM levels of evidence. In: CEBM. https://www.cebm.net/2016/05/ocebm-levels-of-evidence/. Accessed 17 Apr 2020
2. Aromataris E, Munn Z (eds) (2017) Joanna Briggs Institute reviewer's manual. The Joanna Briggs Institute, Adelaide
3. Daly J, Willis K, Small R et al (2007) A hierarchy of evidence for assessing qualitative health research. J Clin Epidemiol 60:43–49. https://doi.org/10.1016/j.jclinepi.2006.03.014
4. EQUATOR Network (2020) What is a reporting guideline?—The EQUATOR Network. https://www.equator-network.org/about-us/what-is-a-reporting-guideline/. Accessed 7 Mar 2020
5. Tong A, Sainsbury P, Craig J (2007) Consolidated criteria for reporting qualitative research (COREQ): a 32-item checklist for interviews and focus groups. Int J Qual Health Care 19:349–357. https://doi.org/10.1093/intqhc/mzm042
6. von Elm E, Altman DG, Egger M et al (2007) The strengthening the reporting of observational studies in epidemiology (STROBE) statement: guidelines for reporting observational studies. PLoS Med 4:e296. https://doi.org/10.1371/journal.pmed.0040296
7. Brouwers MC, Kerkvliet K, Spithoff K, AGREE Next Steps Consortium (2016) The AGREE reporting checklist: a tool to improve reporting of clinical practice guidelines. BMJ 352:i1152. https://doi.org/10.1136/bmj.i1152
8. Moher D, Liberati A, Tetzlaff J et al (2009) Preferred reporting items for systematic reviews and meta-analyses: the PRISMA statement. PLoS Med 6:e1000097. https://doi.org/10.1371/journal.pmed.1000097
9. Boutron I, Page MJ, Higgins JPT, Altman DG, Lundh A, Hróbjartsson A (2019) Chapter 7: Considering bias and conflicts of interest among the included studies. In: Higgins JPT, Thomas J, Chandler J, Cumpston M, Li T, Page MJ, Welch VA (eds). Cochrane Handbook for Systematic Reviews of Interventions version 6.0 (updated July 2019), Cochrane. https://www.training.cochrane.org/handbook
10. Critical Appraisal Skills Programme (2018) CASP checklists. In: CASP—critical appraisal skills programme. https://casp-uk.net/casp-tools-checklists/. Accessed 7 Mar 2020
11. Higgins JPT, Savović J, Page MJ et al (2019) Chapter 8: Assessing risk of bias in a randomized trial. In: Higgins JPT, Thomas J, Chandler J et al (eds) Cochrane handbook for systematic reviews of interventions version 6.0 (updated July 2019). Cochrane, London

12. Guyatt GH, Oxman AD, Kunz R et al (2011) GRADE guidelines 6. Rating the qual-
    ity of evidence—imprecision. J Clin Epidemiol 64:1283–1293. https://doi.org/10.1016/j.
    jclinepi.2011.01.012
13. Sterne JAC, Savović J, Page MJ et al (2019) RoB 2: a revised tool for assessing risk of bias in
    randomised trials. BMJ 366:l4898. https://doi.org/10.1136/bmj.l4898
14. Sterne JA, Hernán MA, Reeves BC et al (2016) ROBINS-I: a tool for assessing risk of bias in
    non-randomised studies of interventions. BMJ 355:i4919. https://doi.org/10.1136/bmj.i4919
15. Wells GA, Shea B, O'Connell D et al (2019) The Newcastle-Ottawa Scale (NOS) for assessing
    the quality of nonrandomised studies in meta-analyses. Ottawa Hospital Research Institute,
    Ottawa. http://www.ohri.ca/programs/clinical_epidemiology/oxford.asp. Accessed 7 Mar 2020
16. Cochrane Community (2020) Glossary—Cochrane community. https://community.cochrane.
    org/glossary#letter-R. Accessed 8 Mar 2020
17. Messick S (1989) Meaning and values in test validation: the science and ethics of assessment.
    Educ Res 18:5–11. https://doi.org/10.3102/0013189X018002005
18. Sparkes AC (2001) Myth 94: qualitative health researchers will agree about validity. Qual
    Health Res 11:538–552. https://doi.org/10.1177/104973230101100409
19. Aguinis H, Solarino AM (2019) Transparency and replicability in qualitative research: the
    case of interviews with elite informants. Strat Manag J 40:1291–1315. https://doi.org/10.1002/
    smj.3015
20. Lincoln YS, Guba EG (1985) Naturalistic inquiry. Sage Publications, Beverly Hills, CA
21. Hannes K (2011) Chapter 4: Critical appraisal of qualitative research. In: Noyes J, Booth
    A, Hannes K et al (eds) Supplementary guidance for inclusion of qualitative research in
    Cochrane systematic reviews of interventions. Cochrane Collaboration Qualitative Methods
    Group, London
22. Munn Z, Porritt K, Lockwood C et al (2014) Establishing confidence in the output of qualita-
    tive research synthesis: the ConQual approach. BMC Med Res Methodol 14:108. https://doi.
    org/10.1186/1471-2288-14-108
23. Toye F, Seers K, Allcock N et al (2013) 'Trying to pin down jelly'—exploring intuitive pro-
    cesses in quality assessment for meta-ethnography. BMC Med Res Methodol 13:46. https://
    doi.org/10.1186/1471-2288-13-46
24. Katikireddi SV, Egan M, Petticrew M (2015) How do systematic reviews incorporate risk
    of bias assessments into the synthesis of evidence? A methodological study. J Epidemiol
    Community Health 69:189–195. https://doi.org/10.1136/jech-2014-204711
25. McKenzie JE, Brennan SE, Ryan RE et al (2019) Chapter 9: Summarizing study char-
    acteristics and preparing for synthesis. In: Higgins JPT, Thomas J, Chandler J et al (eds)
    Cochrane handbook for systematic reviews of interventions version 6.0 (updated July 2019).
    Cochrane, London
26. Deeks JJ, Higgins JPT, Altman DG (2019) Chapter 10: Analysing data and undertaking meta-
    analyses. In: Higgins JPT, Thomas J, Chandler J et al (eds) Cochrane handbook for systematic
    reviews of interventions version 6.0 (updated July 2019). Cochrane, London

Reviewing Quantitative Studies: Meta-analysis and Narrative Approaches

7

Summary Learning Points

- The main methods of analysing quantitative data are the narrative review and meta-analysis.
- Meta-analysis provides a wide range of summary statistics, inducing a weighted pooled estimate, confidence intervals, and heterogeneity statistics.
- There are several important decisions that need to be made if undertaking a meta-analysis, including what data to include, the most appropriate outcome measure, and the meta-analytic model to be used.
- The limitations of statistical testing, in particular the p-value, are important to understand, and the clinical significance should always be considered alongside statistical significance; in most cases it will be more important. Decision-making should never be based on p-values alone.
- Any key decisions can be tested using a sensitivity analysis, which repeats the analysis making different choices.
- If not undertaking a meta-analysis, careful consideration needs to be given regarding presentation of data and how they are to be combined.

There are a number of different options when synthesising quantitative data. Some of the main options are shown in Table 7.1. These range from largely descriptive approaches where transparency in analysis is hard to demonstrate, right through to meta-analysis which combines data from the studies in a way that should be completely transparent and reproducible, which produces a range of summary statistics and provides methods for investigating the data further.

Although simply hearing the word 'statistic' is enough to convince many would-be reviewers to adopt the narrative approach, this has a number of limitations. In particular it does not provide a single summary result, confidence interval or a numeric estimate of heterogeneity which are very important in decision-making. For example, it is difficult to look at a narrative review of studies comparing two treatments for high blood pressure and to say that based on all of the studies that one drug reduced blood pressure by a certain amount more than the other, which is what people reading this sort of review will often want to know. A meta-analysis will do all of this and much more.

E. Purssell, N. McCrae, *How to Perform a Systematic Literature Review*, https://doi.org/10.1007/978-3-030-49672-2_7

Table 7.1 Different methods of synthesising quantitative data [1]

Method of synthesis	Method	Limitations
Narrative review	Describes the results of each study	Not always clear how the relative importance of studies is decided. Conclusions may not be transparent No summary statistic
Summarising effect estimates	Contains information about the results of each study	No clear way of weighting studies No summary statistic
Combining *p*-values	Combines statistical information from each study where there may be limited information	No information on the size of the effect *p*-Values are dependent on sample size as well as size of effect
Vote counting	Counts the number of studies with a positive or negative effect	No information on the size of the effect *p*-Values are dependent on sample size as well as size of effect
Meta-analysis	Range of techniques to combine statistics from two or more studies. Produces a full range of summary statistics	Requires papers or authors to provide sufficient information

7.1 Types of Quantitative Research

There are two broad approaches to quantitative research, one where you manipulate an intervention in some way and the other where you don't actually 'do' anything to the participants but instead observe them over time. Randomised and nonrandomised experimental studies are examples of the first of these. In these types of study you compare two or more groups who receive different interventions. Cohort and case-control observational studies are examples of the second. In these types of study, you observe people, some of whom will do something or have an exposure to something, and some of whom will not.

These different types of study are often seen as forming a hierarchy as we discussed in Chap. 5. This is mainly based on their risk of bias, with randomised studies generally having a lower risk of bias than nonrandom or observational studies. In most cases prospective data collection is also better than retrospective data collection. This is because if you are collecting data prospectively (i.e. as you go along), you have control over the data collection process. With retrospective data you are relying on data that has already been collected, often for quite different purposes. It may have been collected well or it may not have been, but the researcher can't do anything about it.

Throughout this chapter we will be discussing broad principles. Some of these are not directly applicable to all types of research, for example, observational studies are by definition not randomised. However, if you can understand why randomisation is so important, then you will see the issues inherent with nonrandom studies, what can be done about them and why we often moderate our conclusions accordingly.

You may be wondering why we are so concerned about randomisation? There are two main reasons for this. Firstly, random selection of participants and their subsequent random allocation between interventions are two of the main ways of reducing the risk of bias. Secondly, and perhaps more fundamentally, it is important for many statistical tests that we use which rely on the known properties of randomness. The reason for this is that although people often talk about random things as being unpredictable, for example, 'that is so random', actually in the long-term random events are surprisingly predictable. Just think about all of the small things that have to occur for your morning train to run on time for example. There are lots of opportunities for random events to spoil your day, and on any given day, you normally don't know that any of them is going to happen until they occur. But what you do know is that over your whole lifetime of journeys, most of them don't occur on most days. Therefore on a daily basis, randomness may be unpredictable, but over a longer period, it is very predictable. It is this predictability that underlines many of the statistical tests that we use.

7.2   The Logic of Quantitative Research

Some of the challenges that occur with quantitative research become clear if you think about how a researcher might approach a quantitative problem. Often as a researcher you start off with a clinical problem in an individual or group of patients, with let's say asthma. These people are conceptualised as coming from a wider population of people with the same condition. However, we don't normally study populations directly. This may be for practical reasons, such as the population size being too large or too spread out for us to be able to use the whole population; but there are also statistical reasons for not doing so. What we do instead is to take a sample from the population and conduct our research on that sample. We then take the result from the sample and apply it to the population and then from the population back to our patient or patients.

You will notice here a number of what can only be described as 'inferential leaps. First we assume that our patients actually belong to the population that we think they do, but in reality they may not. For example, our patients may have a particular comorbidity alongside their asthma that makes them different to other people with asthma, or our clinic might be particularly good, so our treatment is different to other clinics treating people with asthma. Both of these might have the effect of making our sample a subpopulation or maybe even a completely different population to others with asthma. Secondly we must assume that the sample which we end up adequately represents the population. Here the key is random sampling. The next inferential leaps are that our result adequately reflects the phenomenon that we wanted to measure in the sample; these are issues of validity and reliability; and then that the result from the sample accurately reflects the result that we would get in the population. Finally, if all of this is good, we then assume the result applies to our patients, which is where we started to begin with. As you can see, there are a lot of assumptions and so there is quite a lot that can go wrong.

This process of generalising from sample to population and then back to individuals requires the use of what we refer to as inferential statistics. This term reflects that fact that we are literally making inferences about a population and then individual patients based on our sample data. The ability to take data from one sample and apply it to other groups, settings and times is referred to as generalisability or external validity. After all when you select a sample and undertake research on them as we did in our hypothetical study above, you are not really interested in that sample at all but rather what they tell you about the population from which they are drawn and the individual patients in this population. The sample statistic is thus used to estimate a population value, a value statisticians call a parameter [2]. Incidentally you may think that this is a somewhat old reference; actually Fisher was terribly important and is often thought of as being the 'father of statistics' developing as he did many of the theories that we use today, his most important legacy probably being the p-value. The book from which this reference comes was actually first published in 1925; you can buy copies of later editions quite cheaply, and it is an interesting read.

Not all statistics that you read in a paper are inferential. You will also find descriptive statistics. These are there, as the name suggests, to describe your sample. You may be interested in how your sample compares to the population of interest, and in the case of an RCT, you would definitely be interested in how similar the groups are at the start of the study. Another important set of descriptive statistics are those showing the flow of participants through the study: how many started the study and how many completed it and what happened to those who did not? You may also hear people talk about per-protocol and intention to treat analyses. Per-protocol means that only those participants who followed the treatment plan exactly would be analysed, whereas intention to treat analyses everyone who was randomised whether or not they followed the treatment plan [3]. Intention to treat analyses are the most common today, as the reasons for participants not following their allotted treatment may be important. You may also hear 'rules of thumb' about what proportion of participants can be lost before this damages the validity of a study. It is not the number that is important, although that may suggest something about the intervention, but the reasons for this loss. If they have moved house, that is a somewhat different situation to if they have had nasty side effects that led to their leaving the study.

We suggest a four-stage approach to understanding the results in quantitative papers based on Fisher's three purposes of statistics: the study of populations, the study of variation and the study of methods of the reduction of data, which is concerned with finding the relevant information in the data.

1. Point estimate of the effect size—this is what people normally think of as being 'the result. It will be a single number such as a mean or median blood pressure, the odds or risk of dying, etc. The 'point' of point estimate refers to the fact that it is a single number, and the 'estimate' part refers to the fact that as long as the sample is adequately selected from the population, and randomly allocated between any interventions being studied, this should be an unbiased estimate of the population parameter. An effect size is simply the amount of something, in this case whatever the study is measuring.

2. Measure of variability or uncertainty—this shows how much variation there is in the data or the precision of the point estimate as an estimate of the population parameter. For the data in the study, it might be a standard deviation or interquartile range and for the estimate of the population parameter a standard error. This may also be expressed as a confidence interval.

3. Clinical significance—this is your judgement, it really is the answer to the question 'does the result matter?' This is where you demonstrate to your reader (or marker!) your expertise in the subject because it is the application of the data to your question. We will talk about this more when discussing GRADE in Chap. 9 as this will help you to decide if a particular set of results is clinically significant or not and some of the principles can be applied to individual studies as well.

4. Measure of statistical significance (p-value)—this is purposely last even though it is often the first thing that people look for. Of all of these numbers, it is probably the least important, as the p-value has a more limited meaning than many people think. It is not the probability that the hypothesis/null hypothesis is true or the probability that the result has occurred by chance; instead it answers the somewhat less interesting question 'what is the probability of getting this result, or one more extreme, given that the null hypothesis is true?' We will return to this later.

To understand how this looks in a paper, let us consider a study by Sherman et al. [4], who undertook some research that may be of interest to students everywhere, attempting to answer the question *does caffeine improve memory*? After drinking caffeinated or decaffeinated coffee, college-age adults completed a range of memory tasks in both the early morning and late afternoon. Here we look at the results for cued recall, defined as the proportion of study words correctly recalled (the paper says percentage, but we have confirmed with the authors that they really are proportions). They report:

- *Follow-up t-tests illustrated that participants who ingested caffeinated coffee (M = 0.44, SD = 0.13) performed better than those who drank decaffeinated coffee (M = 0.34, SD = 0.13) on cued recall, t(58) = 2.90, p < 0.01, Cohen's d = 0.75, CI [0.22,1.27].*

In this sentence the researchers are telling you that the mean score in the caffeine group was 0.44, and in the decaffeinated group, it was 0.34, a difference of 0.1. We actually have three-point estimates of effect sizes here, the single numbers that summarise the results in each group and the difference between the groups which is what we are really interested in. The next thing that you want to know is how spread out the scores were, and you can see that in both groups the standard deviation was 0.13, so the spread of results was very similar in both groups. These numbers are both measurements of the group means, mean difference and dispersion in the sample (and so are descriptive); and an estimate of the same values in the population (and so are inferential). You must ask yourself, do you think that this is a clinically significant difference?; does this difference of 0.1 matter? We have now looked at steps 1–3.

The next section is the test of statistical significance; it says that they used a t-test, with 58 degrees of freedom, which gave a p-value of <0.01. Using the traditional 'rules' of statistical testing and the null hypothesis significance test in particular, we would say based on this p-value that the result is statistically significant.

7.3   More About p-values

It is worth spending a little time on the p-value because it is often the first (and sometimes the only) detail sought by readers, and it is widely misunderstood. It is defined as the probability of getting the data (or data more extreme) if the null hypothesis is assumed to be true. It is dependent on sample size; exactly the same result with a larger or smaller sample will produce a different p-value. Many statistical tests also make an assumption that the sample has been randomly selected from the population and once selected that individuals are randomly allocated to the different treatments or interventions being tested. In practice many samples in healthcare research are not randomly selected from the population, and people tend not to worry as much as they should about this. The other name for a random sample is a 'probability sample', so called because everyone in the population has a known and equal probability of being in the sample.

You may hear nonrandom samples referred to as 'convenience samples'. This maybe problematic for most statistical tests that assume random sampling, and you should look carefully at the selection process for signs of bias. However, even when studies do have random samples, they are often not really random samples of the whole population of interest. Take, for example, a study of people with asthma that is conducted in London. You might logically conclude that people with asthma are one big worldwide population, and so data from a sample in one country can be applied in another. This may sound extreme, but we do this all of the time on a smaller scale when we apply research in one country that has been undertaken in a different country. Probability or random sampling assumes that everyone in the population has a known and equal probability of being in the sample; in this case of course, they do not. Someone with asthma in New York has zero probability of being in a random sample recruited in London, for example. The dilemma here was summarised nicely by Fisher, when he said 'The postulate of randomness thus resolves itself into the question, 'Of what population is this a random sample?'' [5, p. 313].

The p-value is most commonly used as part of the null hypothesis significance test, which is surprisingly complex, consisting of a number of stages:

- Start with a hypothesis that you believe may be true; this is sometimes called the alternative or research hypothesis to differentiate it from the null hypothesis. This is your hypothesis.
- Flip this to become a null hypothesis, which will often (but not always) be the direct opposite of the hypothesis; this is the thing that the *p*-value assumes is true. The important thing here is that you do not really believe this hypothesis, it is simply there to be refuted or not.
- Collect your data.
- Calculate the probability of getting the data that you collected, or data more extreme, if you believe that the null hypothesis that you constructed above is correct—this is the *p*-value. Note that you are using the null hypothesis here that you really do not believe anyway, not the hypothesis that you do actually believe.
- If the *p*-value is very low, it means the probability of getting your results (or results more extreme) if the null hypothesis is true is also very low, suggesting one of them is wrong. As a researcher you hope your results are true; if they are not, we best all go home! By convention, 'very low' in this context is taken to mean a probability of <0.05 or 5%. This figure is another legacy or Fisher, but it is just convention; you can change it.
- Presuming that you believe your data *are* right, you must therefore conclude that the null hypothesis is false, so you reject the null hypothesis and accept the opposite alternative hypothesis. This may seem odd at first, but the logic is that if the null hypothesis is likely to be wrong, then its alternative hypothesis is likely to be right.
- Your original (alternative) hypothesis, therefore, is supported by the data, although crucially never tested directly.

In this case the *p*-value is less than 0.01, meaning the probability of getting this result or one more extreme with a sample size of 60, if we assume that the null hypothesis of no difference between the groups to be true is less than 1%, well below the normal cutoff of 0.05 or 5%. We therefore conclude that the data do not support the null hypothesis of no difference, which we can therefore reject in favour of the alternative hypothesis that there is a real difference between the groups. Remember though, although the data do seem to support the alternative hypothesis, we have never actually tested this directly; we only conclude this because the data are incompatible with the null hypothesis.

A warning should be given here. The *p*-value is probably the most misunderstood entity in statistics. The American Statistical Association recently gave guidance about *p*-values [6], noting in particular that:

1. They do not measure the probability that the hypothesis is true or the probability that the data were produced by chance alone.
2. Decisions about the results of a study should not be based only on whether a *p*-value is <0.05 or any other arbitrary figure.
3. They do not measure effect or show the importance of the result.

Guidance in the *Statistical Analyses and Methods in the Published Literature* (SAMPL) guideline [7] states that *p*-values should be reported exactly; in the past, *p*-values of 0.05 or more were often reported simply as 'not significant, and all values of less than 0.05 reported thus <0.05. One other thing, you can't have a *p*-value of 0.000; if your software reports it, what it usually means is <0.0005, and this is normally reported in journals as being <0.001. You may also see them identified as p values, p-values, P values, and P-values. Here we use *p*-value which is in keeping with the American Statistical Association guidance referred to above.

7.3.1 Why the *p*-value Is Not the Probability That the Result Is Due to Chance, and the Probability of Getting Your Result May Be Zero

One thing that we often hear about the *p*-value is that it is the probability that the result has occurred by chance. This is wrong. As it is such a widespread misconception, it is worth just getting your head around why this is not the case and why it *cannot* be the case. You will recall that the null hypothesis significance test is based on rejecting or not rejecting the null hypothesis. You will also recall that the null hypothesis essentially states that there is no real effect, and so any effect that you do see is the result of chance. In our example it would state that there is no difference between those consuming caffeine and those not; and any difference that we do see is not real but has occurred by chance. Therefore, if we retain the null hypothesis, this is saying the result *is* due to chance, and if the result *is* due to chance, the probability of it being the result of chance is 1 or 100%. Something that is true has a probability of 100%.

If on the other hand the *p*-value is below the rejection level, typically <0.05, then we reject the null hypothesis. If we reject the null hypothesis, then we are saying that the probability that this has occurred by chance is zero, as we are saying the null hypothesis is not true. Something that is not true has a probability of 0%. The important point is that under the null hypothesis significance test, the probability that the result has occurred by chance can only be 1 (if we retain the null hypothesis) or 0 (if we reject it) [8].

When analysing continuous data, you might also be surprised to know that the probability of getting any specific numeric result is extremely small, even if it is the same as the result that you got from your study. To understand why, imagine taking the blood pressures of ten people all of whom had a blood pressure of 120/80 mmHg. How many of your sample had a blood pressure of 120/80 mmHg? The answer of course is none of them; we use these numbers as approximations, 120 mmHg may actually mean 119.5–120.4 mmHg, for example. It is extremely unlikely that anyone has a blood pressure of *exactly* 120 mmHg. This is why we don't talk about the *p*-value as the probability of getting our result but rather the probability of getting our result *or one more extreme*.

If you are finding all of this difficult to take in and to make sense of, perhaps this quote from statistician Matt Briggs might reassure you. When discussing this very subject, he wrote: 'the p value, a probability concept so misaligned with intuition that no civilian can hold it firmly in mind (nor, judging by what finds its way into textbooks, can more than a few statisticians)' [9, p. 30]. Incidentally, having said that the *p*-value does not test the hypothesis directly, you may be wondering if you can? The answer is yes you can, using a branch of statistics known as Bayesian analysis. We will say no more about this here, but there are plenty of resources about this online.

7.4 Statistical Errors

There are two types of statistical error that are possible with p-values: a Type I error is rejecting the null hypothesis when it is true (this is finding a difference when really there is not one—you might think of this as a 'false positive' result); while a Type II error is failing to reject the null hypothesis when it is false (failing to find a difference when there really is one—a 'false negative' result). The relationship between these is shown in Table 7.2. Type II errors often occur because of sample sizes that are too small; the technical term for this is that they are underpowered, which is one of the rationales for undertaking meta-analysis—we will return to this later! Incidentally one of the favourite conclusions of students and researchers alike is 'more and bigger studies'. This is not right, just as studies that are too small run a risk of making a Type II error; studies that are too large run the risk of making a Type I error—finding erroneous statistically significant relationships. What we want is really 'more and appropriately sized' studies. To do this we undertake a power analysis to calculate the sample size needed. Don't worry too much about how this is done; as a reviewer what you are really interested in is how the authors have decided on their sample size. If they have done a power analysis which will calculate the right sample size, this is a good sign. One very simple way to minimise the risk of making spurious statistical decisions is to not worry so much about the p-value and instead to concentrate on the results—ask yourself 'does this result matter?'

We often find that students are confused by this process and the slightly odd meaning of the p-value. It is confusing; our advice is to know it and not worry too much about why it is what it is. It just is. If you like rhymes, you might find it helpful to think of it this way: *if the p is low, the null must go*. A second line could be *if the null does go, the alternative must be so*.

In the study by Sherman et al. [4], that we referred to previously, the paper also gave a statistic called Cohen's *d*. This is a standardised mean difference, that is, a difference between the two means expressed not in the original unit of measurement but in a number of standard deviations; thus there is a difference of 0.75 standard

Table 7.2 Types of statistical error

	The null hypothesis is *really* true	The null hypothesis is *really* false
Based on our *results*, we don't reject the null hypothesis (the p-value is *not* <0.05)	*Correctly* failed to reject the null hypothesis—there is no real difference which you correctly identified (the probability of this is $1 - \alpha$)	*Type II error* incorrectly failed to reject the null hypothesis (the probability of this known as β)
Based on our *results*, we do reject the null hypothesis (the p-value *is* <0.05)	*Type I error* incorrectly rejecting the null hypothesis (the probability of this is known as α)	*Correctly* rejected the null hypothesis—there is a real difference which you correctly identified (the probability of this is $= 1 - \beta$, or the power of the study)

deviations between the two groups (if you identified this as a point estimate of an effect size, well done!). We go into much more detail about what this means in the next section. The confidence interval here (which is the measure of dispersion) is saying that if this study were repeated many times, 95% of the confidence intervals calculated from these replications, of which this is one, would contain the true population value. It is *not* really correct to say that this is the range within which we can be 95% sure that the population value lies; that is the definition of the credible interval which is something very different. Like the *p*-value conventional confidence intervals like this have a slightly odd meaning.

You may wonder how it is you can take data from sometimes quite a small sample, in this case only 60 participants, and apply it to a much broader population. As long as the sample is randomly selected and allocated between the two groups, the study result will provide what is known as an *unbiased estimate* of the equivalent parameter in the population. However, because you only have one sample from an infinite number of samples that could be drawn from the population, we need to work out how much that result might vary if you had a different sample to the one that you actually did recruit? After all, the sample is 'accidental' in as much as it is a random sample; and a sample of Bob, Emily and Sally will give a slightly different result to a sample containing Bob, Emily and Joe. If we did repeat this study many times, each time caclulating a result this would provide a 'distribution' of results, reflecting the individual differences between people in different samples. The variation in point estimates that result from the theoretical distribution associated with different samples is captured in a number known as the standard error and its associated confidence interval.

All this talk of standard errors and deviations is a bit confusing; the most important thing is not to get them mixed up; the standard error is always smaller than the standard deviation. These are explained more in Box 7.1.

Before we move on, there is one final issue to discuss about randomisation. While it is crucial to many statistical tests, it cannot do the two things that most people want, which is to make the sample representative of the population and the experimental and control groups the same. It does reduce the risk of bias, but if you think about it for a minute by definition, randomisation can't ensure anything—it is random! It is also important to note that some study designs make random sampling difficult or practically impossible. We are not saying that these are worthless, juat that they are inherently more susceptible to bias.

Box 7.1 Standard Deviations v Standard Errors
Both are measures of variability. The standard deviation reflects the variability in the sample, which you may recall will also therefore tell you about the variability of individual results in the population. The standard error refers the variation in point estimates of the effect size that you would get if you were to repeat the study many, many times, each time with a slightly different random sample. Now of course you are not going to do that, so it is a theoretical number that is calculated from the standard deviation like this: $SE = SD/\sqrt{(sample\ size)}$. The standard error is therefore a standard deviation, but not of individual data points (that is the standard deviation!) but of the summary point estimate values. It can be thought of as reflecting the precision of the point estimate [10].

To summarise, there are four elements in understanding the result of a quantitative study:

1. Point estimate of the effect size—a single number.
2. Measure of variability—a range of numbers.
3. Clinical significance—your opinion about whether it matters.
4. Measure of statistical significance—the *p*-value.

7.5   Introducing Meta-analysis

Meta-analysis is the statistical aggregation and analysis of data from multiple studies to produce a combined result. The term was coined by educationalist Gene Glass:

> 'Meta-analysis refers to the analysis of analyses. I use it to refer to the statistical analysis of a large collection of analysis results from individual studies for the purpose of integrating the findings. It connotes a rigorous alternative to the casual, narrative discussions of research studies'. [11, p. 3]

A demonstration of the value of meta-analysis in healthcare research was given by Lau et al. [12], who investigated the effect on mortality of streptokinase versus a placebo for patients with acute myocardial infarction. Although many (but not all) of the older studies showed that the treatment reduced mortality, their small sample sizes made the results very variable and in most cases statistically insignificant due to the resultant very wide confidence intervals. It turned out that these studies were underpowered, that is, they were making Type II errors because of their small sample sizes. Remember a Type II error is when you fail to reject a null hypothesis when you really should. However, when the results of studies were aggregated on a cumulative basis, that is, each time a new study is published, it is added on to those done before; the beneficial effect of the treatment was clear as far back as 1973—15 years before the last study in the meta-analysis. Researchers continued with studies long after the evidence already existed that the treatment worked, but nobody had performed the necessary meta-analysis on the existing data that would have shown this, thus missing the potentially lifesaving conclusion that these drugs reduced mortality.

However, undertaking meta-analysis entails more than simply averaging study results or counting the number of studies that reach particular conclusions. For a result to be accurate, other factors should be considered such as the contribution that each study should make to this overall result and different assumptions about the nature of the data. We will discuss these later. The process is of undertaking a meta-analysis is as follows:

1. Extract the data of interest from each study.
2. Calculate a pooled estimate of the effect in the form of a weighted average of all of the studies, including a confidence interval showing the precision of this point estimate. These are equivalent to the point estimate and measure of variability to which we referred earlier.

3. Calculate a p-value to assess the statistical significance of the result.
4. Assess the heterogeneity of the results, showing whether the variation in results between the studies included in the meta-analysis is suggestive of real differences in the true effect that each study is estimating or whether any variation is attributable to sampling error alone. This step is sometimes omitted, in which case one is undertaking a fixed-effects model analysis.
5. Other techniques and plots, such as meta-regression and subgroup analysis, and forest and funnel plots may be used to display and analyse patterns in the data.

From now on, for clarity we will differentiate between the data extracted from each study and the *pooled effect size* and its confidence interval, which is the weighted average effect from all of the studies together—that is, the point estimate of the effect size in the meta-analysis. If you are confused by all of these effect sizes, try Box 7.2 which explains them all in one place.

Box 7.2 Effect Sizes

Effect size, standardised effect size and pooled effect size. What a lot of effect sizes! The effect size is the thing that you are measuring, usually in the unit in which you are measuring it, for example, a difference in blood pressure in mmHg, life expectancy in years and distance in miles. These are sometimes referred to as 'raw' effect sizes. In the case of a meta-analysis, each study will contribute at least one effect size, and you will also calculate a pooled effect size. The p-value is not an effect size because it varies according to sample size—you cannot directly compare two p-values.

Standardised effect sizes have the unit of measurement removed; this is the process known as standardisation. In most cases this is done by dividing the effect size by its standard deviation, thus turning the raw effect size into a number of standard deviations. In the case of a difference between two means, it would be the mean in one group minus the mean in the other group, which is then divided by the standard deviation. There are three ways of doing this: Cohen's d which uses the pooled standard deviation of both groups as the denominator; Glass' Δ which uses the standard deviation of the control group only; and Hedges' g which is very similar to Cohen's d but contains a correction for small sample sizes. You use a standardised effect size rather than a 'raw' effect size if the studies are measuring the same thing but in different ways that cannot easily be converted to be the same. Many other statistics can be converted to be a standardised effect size which can be very useful if studies report the data differently.

Finally the pooled effect size is a number of effect sizes combined by calculating a weighted average. The pooled effect size can be of ordinary effect sizes or of standardised effect sizes. It will also have a p-value, but remember that the p-value is not an effect size as it can't be compared between studies. The pooled effect size is also normally used as a point estimate of a population parameter.

Table 7.3 Data that needs to be extracted for meta-analysis

Type of data	Data to be extracted
Correlation	Correlation coefficient and the sample size
Dichotomous	Number of events and number of observations in each group
Mean difference	Mean, standard deviation and sample size for each group. Note it is the standard deviation and not the standard error
Proportions	The number of events and number of observations

7.6   Extracting the Data

The first task when conducting the actual meta-analysis is to identify and extract the summary data from each study. The exact data needed will for a meta-analysis will depend on your question and the nature of the summary statistics in the paper; some examples are given in Table 7.3. The best way of arranging these data are in a spreadsheet; examples are given in Appendix A: *How to do a Meta-analysis*.

7.7   Calculate a Pooled Estimate of the Effect

The first decision here it to work out what your summary effect size should be. The effect measure that you use will depends on the review question, the type of data in the studies and what you think will make sense. For analysis of continuous data with the mean as its outcome, you could use the raw mean difference (simply the difference between the two means) or the standardised mean difference (the difference between two means divided by the standard deviation). A standardised effect size is necessary if studies used different methods of measuring the effect, as the process of standardising data removes the unit of measurement and so makes them comparable. Sometimes it is easy to convert data to the same scale (e.g. Fahrenheit and centigrade) which you should do if you can as measurement scales are important. There are different ways of calculating standardised mean differences, including Cohen's *d*, Glass' *Δ* and Hedges' *g* [13], but generally the differences are not usually important, and a meta-analysis programme will use one of these by default. If studies have dichotomous data, you could use the odds or risk ratios, risk difference or number needed to treat/harm. It is always important to consider what would make most sense to the reader; relative changes can be hard to interpret (a 200% of not very much is probably not very much), so many people prefer absolute differences instead. This is the equivalent of saying 'carrots have gone up in price by 20 pence' which is an absolute increase rather than the relative 'carrots have gone up in price by 15%'.

Many other statistics can also be analysed, including single proportions and before and after results. For a comprehensive list, you can look in the manual for the R [14] package *metafor* [15] which goes into some detail about this and gives some useful advice about them. Some of these require transformation prior to analysis to fulfil the assumptions of the techniques used, for example, taking the log of the odds ratio and relative risk and Fisher's r to z transformation for correlations. Although this may seem daunting, the transformation process is usually done by the meta-analysis programme, but you should be aware of what is happening to the data.

It is possible to standardise a large number of different statistics by converting among them, including p-values and correlation coefficients. Among the tools that can do this are the R package *compute.es* [16] and online calculators such as that provided by the Campbell Collaboration (https://campbellcollaboration.org/effect-size-calculato.html).

7.7.1   Interpreting Standardised Effect Sizes

Standardised effect sizes which are expressed in standard deviations can be difficult to interpret; what does the result *Cohen's d = 0.75, CI [0.22,1.27]* given above mean, for example? A rule of thumb is that a standardised mean difference of 0.2 is a small effect, 0.5 a moderate effect, and 0.8 a large effect [17]. Sawilowsky [18] graded standardised mean differences as 0.01 = very small, 0.2 = small, 0.5 = medium, 0.8 = large, 1.2 = very large, and 2.0 = huge. These are not rules, though. If you look back at our example earlier, you can hopefully now interpret the findings of the coffee study which provided results in Cohen's d as being a moderate or medium to large effect.

7.8   Vote Counting

Before actually pooling the data, let us consider an alternative known as vote counting, which simply compares the number of studies with positive and negative outcomes. Although there are formal techniques for vote counting [19], there are fundamental problems with the way that approach is often implemented. It is not always straightforward to decide whether a result counts as being positive or negative. For example, does a nonstatistically significant but positive result count, or does it have to have a p-value of <0.05? Statistical significance may be used, but this is prone to the limitations of p-values discussed previously. Vote counting also does not easily allow for differential weighting of studies; large and small studies are often counted equally which could lead to a situation where two studies of ten participants each showing a negative effect takes precedence over one study of 10,000 participants with a positive result. It also does not provide summary statistics, confidence intervals or estimates of heterogeneity. The question that vote counting most satisfactorily answers is the fairly broad question 'Is there any evidence of an effect?' [1] which is somewhat less interesting than the question a meta-analysis will provide an answer to.

7.9   Models of Meta-analysis

If you want to do a meta-analysis, one of the early decisions you must make is to decide on the model of analysis to be used. There are two main models, the fixed and random-effects models. To understand why there is more than one, consider a meta-analysis of four studies investigating a treatment for hypertension. Each study has a result which we refer to as the observed effect, which we use to estimate the true effect in the population. This is precisely the same process that we discussed at the beginning of this chapter, an observed effect in the study estimating true effect in the population. Earlier we referred to them as a statistic and a parameter, respectively; here we are going to refer to them as the observed and true effects.

Each study in the meta-analysis will provide an observed effect, which are likely to vary as each study will have a different result. This variation may be accounted for in two ways:

1. The studies are estimating the same true underlying effect, and so the observed results differ due to sampling error alone, that is, the study results are not really different; they just appear to be so because the participants in the studies are different. This is known as the fixed-effects model.
2. The studies are estimating different but related true underlying effects, as such they differ due to both sampling error and differences in the underlying true effects. This is known as the random-effects model.

An interesting fact about the fixed-effects model is that as it assumes any variation in results is due to sampling error alone; it follows that if the studies had infinitely large sample sizes and thus no sampling error, they would produce exactly the same results. The fixed-effects model therefore makes conditional inferences about the pooled effect estimate based only on the studies in the meta-analysis [20]. The fixed part of the name refers to the fact that the underlying true effect being estimated is literally 'fixed' accross the studies.

The random-effects model makes what appears to be a more realistic assumption, which is that although the studies are similar (hence their inclusion in the meta-analysis), it is not assumed that they are measuring exactly the same underlying true effect. A drug may be unchanged from one study to another, but each experiment will be conducted in different places, at different times and by different people. So instead of a single true underlying effect, the random-effects model assumes a distribution of true effect sizes of which our studies are considered to be only a sample.

The effect of this is that the result of a random-effects meta-analysis contains two sources of variation, the variation due to sampling error within each study which was described above and the variation between studies that occurs because they are not measuring exactly the same true effect. The between-studies variation is captured in its standard deviation, represented by a figure known as τ (this is the Greek letter 'Tau'), although you will commonly see the between-studies variance τ^2 (Tau^2) given. This number is one of a range of numbers which are collectively known as heterogeneity statistics. We will return to these later, for now it is enough to know that this model allows for variation caused by sampling error just as the fixed-effects model does *and* because the true effects being estimated differ, which the fixed-effects model does not. The random-effects model, therefore, makes inferences beyond the studies in the meta-analysis to all of the studies that have or could be done [20].

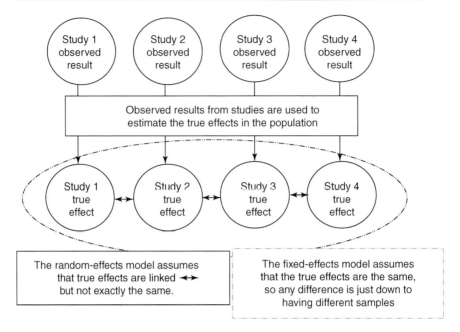

Fig. 7.1 Fixed and random-effects model

These models are shown in Fig. 7.1, where the circles at the top are the observed study results. At the bottom we have the true but unknown effects in the population which are the same in the fixed-effects model (dotted circle) but not in the random-effects model where they are related but different (arrows).

7.10   Weighting

We have said previously that the main output of a meta-analysis is a weighted average pooled effect size, which means that the studies are weighted so that some studies contribute more to the final result than others. This seems fair; a very large study should contribute more to the result than a very small study. In the fixed-effects model, the weighting that is applied is simply the inverse of each studies variance (that is 1/study variance), while in the random-effects model, it is the inverse of each studies variance *plus* the between studies variance (1/study variance + τ^2). Because each studies variance is proportional to sample size (larger samples lead to smaller variances), using the inverse of variance ensures that these larger studies are more heavily weighted than their smaller equivalents. The addition of τ^2, the within-studies variance to the random-effects model means that the weighting of each study in this model is less affected by its sample size, and so the weights tend to be more balanced. This is because the τ^2 element is the same across all of the studies. Fixed-effects models will therefore amplify the differences between larger and smaller studies which may be interesting in itself. You may hear this referred to as 'small study effects'.

7.11   Assess the Heterogeneity of the Results

Heterogeneity, which when used in a general way refers to diversity within a particular group or setting, is a major consideration in meta-analysis as it should be in any systematic review. There are three main sources of heterogeneity in a systematic review [21], these being:

1. Clinical heterogeneity or diversity which refers to variation in patients, treatments and outcomes
2. Methodological heterogeneity or diversity which arises from differences in study design and conduct
3. Statistical heterogeneity which refers to differences in study results

The reviewer should attend to the first two of these types of heterogeneity at an early stage, ensuring that studies fulfil eligibility criteria. The results of a meta-analysis are really concerned with last of these, statistical heterogeneity. This occurs when the results of the individual studies vary more than would be expected from chance or random error alone [21]. Although there are these three sources of heterogeneity, in practice if you hear the term heterogeneity referred to in a meta-analysis, it is always statistical heterogeneity.

Statistical heterogeneity may be assessed in a two-step process:

1. The first question is whether there is statistically significant heterogeneity. This is primarily answered by Cochran's Q test, which is calculated by adding the weighted squared deviations between each study result and the pooled effect estimate. The result of this test is then compared to the χ^2 distribution, with the degrees of freedom (the number of studies -1) to give a p-value. Whenever you have a p-value you must be clear what the null hypothesis is, in this case it is of homogeneity. If the p-value is low, the null hypothesis of homogeneity is rejected, and the alternative hypothesis of heterogeneity is accepted. A p-value of <0.1 rather than the more common <0.05 is generally used for this decision, due to the limited statistical power of this test [22]. If you don't know what this means, we discuss this issue earlier in the chapter; briefly it means that using a level of 0.05 would sometimes fail to reject this null hypothesis when it should be rejected; therefore it would make a Type II statistical error. You may also hear people refer to this as being an 'underpowered test' for this reason. Importantly the Q test shows whether there is heterogeneity, but not how much (remember a p-value is not an effect size).
2. The extent of heterogeneity is shown by I^2 (the I meaning inconsistency), which shows the percentage of variability in the final result that is due to heterogeneity rather than sampling error.

Although the original authors who developed this statistic warned against 'naive categorisation' of the I^2 statistic output, they presented 'tentative adjectives' to categorise different values. They suggested that an I^2 of 25% would be low heterogeneity, 50% moderate and 75% high [22]. A high level of heterogeneity does not

Table 7.4 Interpretation of I^2 scores

I^2	Interpretation
0–40%	Might not be important
30–60%	May represent moderate heterogeneity
50–90%	May represent substantial heterogeneity
75–100%	Considerable heterogeneity

indicate that a meta-analysis is wrong, but such variation needs explanation. The *Cochrane Handbook* [21] issued the following 'rough guide to interpretation' shown in Table 7.4.

A method of investigating heterogeneity that is less widely used but may be very useful is the calculation of the *prediction interval*. This shows the range of true effect sizes that can be expected in future studies; it literally predicts future studies based on the studies that you have in the review. It has the big advantage of being very intuitive, using the same scale as the studies in the review. If the prediction interval is the same or similar to the confidence interval, there is not evidence of significant heterogeneity; if it is wider, then there may be significant heterogeneity [23]. Finally there are a range of 'leave-one-out' and other influence analyses that look at the effects of each study on the results; these might identify individual studies that are particularly significant in their contribution to any heterogeneity [20].

Heterogeneity is sometimes seen as a 'problem', but like any research result, it should really be seen for what it is, it is part of the result of your review, and it may in itself be an important finding. Satisfactorily explaining it will be an even more important finding. Contrary to what you may see done in practice, it should also not be used as a method of choosing between the fixed and random-effects models; this decision should be made before not after the analysis as the different models make different assumptions and answer different questions. Lastly the absence of statistical heterogeneity does not demonstrate homogeneity in the other areas, after all you can travel by bus, by train, or if you are very wealthy by helicopter. These have homogeneity of outcome (they all lead to you arriving at your destination), but they are very different methods of arrival.

7.12   Investigating Heterogeneity: Subgroup Analysis and Meta-regression

One method of investigating heterogeneity is to undertake subgroup analyses, whereby studies are grouped according to one or more hypothesised moderating or influencing factors. For example, studies conducted in hospital or community settings may be expected to produce different results, and this may justify analysing each of these studies separately as well as together. On the other hand, you may decide that these are two completely different populations in which case you should do separate analyses.

Meta-regression merges the techniques of meta-analysis and regression to investigate the presence and extent of a relationship between the effect sizes in the analysis and one or more moderating factors [24]. For example, you might think that the results of different studies were related to the year of publication, for example if you think treatements have improved over time, you could do a meta-regression of the results against year. As well as linear predictor variables, categorical independent variables can also be used, just as they can with 'normal' regression. Such an analysis will provide an R^2 value which shows the proportion of total variance that is explained by the regression model and a test for residual heterogeneity which shows whether the remaining heterogeneity after the regression (which takes account of the predictor variables) is more than expected through sampling error alone [20]. The important thing about these methods is that they should really be planned in advance, and if not at the very least make scientific sense. Otherwise you may be accused of 'fishing' for explanations. We discuss this in Chap. 10.

Meta-analysis of individual participant data may also be undertaken. By using each participant as the unit of analysis rather than the study, this approach allows results to be generalised at patient rather than study level. The major difficulty, however, is in getting the raw data from researchers. Unsurprisingly, such analysis is rarely done [25].

7.13   Forest Plots

A forest plot is a graphical display of the results of quantitative studies. This has really become the standard graphical output in meta-analyses [26] and is increasingly being used for other types of study as well. Although forest plots drawn by different programmes look slightly different, they have common features. The forest plot in Fig. 7.2 uses data from a Cochrane Review investigating antibiotics for the

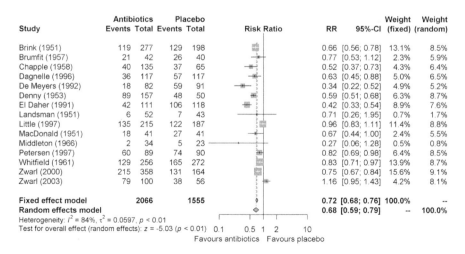

Fig. 7.2 Forest plot of antibiotics versus placebo for treatment of sore throat (outcome: symptom of sore throat on day 3)

treatment of sore throat [27] and was produced by the R package called *meta* [28]. If you want to look at the original plot, you can find it here: https://www.cochraneli-brary.com/cdsr/doi/10.1002/14651858.CD000023.pub4/references#CD000023-fig-00101 and the code to do the analysis is in Appendix A.

Let us explain what this forest plot does:

- Each horizontal line shows the result of one study. So the study by Brink et al. [29] had 119 events out of 227 in the antibiotic group and 129 out of 198 in the placebo group (events being having a sore throat after three days). This gave a risk ratio of 0.66 and a 95% confidence interval of 0.56–0.78.
- The box represents the study result and the size of the box reflects the weighting associated with each study.
- The study results are shown numerically to the left of the plot and the weightings in fixed-effects and random-effects models to the right. As we discussed earlier, there is more variation in the weighting applied to the fixed-effects model.
- The 'line of no difference' or null line is in the middle and shows where results that mean there is no difference between the two groups would lie.
- If the box is to the left of the null line, this favours the experimental group, if it is to the right, it favours the control group; the distance away from the line shows the strength of the result. You may find this reversed, so always check the labels to confirm which way around this is. Although it will be indicated, if you are looking at a difference such as the mean difference or risk difference, that is, one group minus another group, the number that means no difference will be 0; if you are looking at a ratio such as the odds or risk ratio, which is one group divided by another (as we are here), it will be 1 as it is here.
- The horizontal line for each study shows the 95% confidence interval. If the confidence interval touches or crosses the null line, the result however strong (and however clinically significant) is not statistically significant. If you are not sure what a confidence interval is, we discussed this at the beginning of this chapter.
- The pooled effect size in both fixed-effects and random-effects models are shown as diamonds: the centre of the diamond is the summary or pooled effect size, and the edges the confidence interval. This is a convention across meta-analysis programmes, so if you see a diamond, it is always a pooled result. You will also see the pooled effect size given in numbers on the bottom right, and the association *p*-value on the bottom left.
- The heterogeneity statistics I^2 and the Q test *p*-value are shown at the bottom left of the plot just above the test of statistical significance for the overall result.

The pooled risk ratio in this example is 0.68 using the random-effects model, meaning a 32% reduction in the risk that a person has having a sore throat 3 days after starting antibiotic treatment. This is statistically significant because the confidence interval does not include the number that means no difference, which in this case is 1 (it being a risk *ratio*). This is confirmed by the *p*-value for overall effect, which is <0.01, meaning that the probability of getting this result, if the null hypothesis of no difference between the groups is true, is less than 0.01 or 1%. As this is below the accepted threshold of 0.05, the data are not consistent with the null hypothesis of no difference, and therefore we reject this in favour of the alternative hypothesis which is that there is a difference. The heterogeneity p-value is <0.01, meaning that we can similarly reject the null hypothesis of homogeneity in favour of the alternative hypothesis of heterogeneity. Heterogeneity is confirmed by the I^2 value of 84%.

It seems complicated, but actually we are just going to apply the same rules as we did for individual studies:

1. The point estimate of the pooled effect size—in this case it is a risk ratio of 0.68, which equates to a reduction of 32% in the risk of having a sore throat in those taking antibiotics compared to those not.
2. Measure of variability or uncertainty—which is the confidence interval. Look to see how wide it is and whether it touches or crosses that null line. Strictly speaking this is saying that if you repeated this study an infinite number of times, 95% of those replications would include the true value; but as this is confusing, it can be thought of as an estimate of the precision of the result. You also need to consider the heterogeneity associated with the result here as these may add to any uncertainty about the result.
3. Clinical significance—this would include the point estimate and heterogeneity statistics above. Do you think that a reduction of 32% is important? What about a reduction of 32% where 84% of that result can be accounted for by heterogeneity?
4. Measure of statistical significance (p-value)—are the data consistent with the null hypothesis of no difference or not? If not you reject the null hypothesis of no difference and conclude that the alternative hypothesis of a difference is probably correct. You will know this both by the p-value itself, is it less than the cutoff of 0.05?; and by the confidence interval, if it touches or crosses the null line the result will not be statistically significant.

7.14   Publication Bias and Funnel Plots

Publication bias is sometimes an overlooked problem in healthcare research. It occurs when authors or editors make decisions regarding the publication of study results on the basis of the strength or direction of the studies' findings [30]. Any influence apart from scientific rigour on the decision whether to publish a study is suggestive of publication bias. It is perhaps easier than ever before to search data that have not been published in traditional journals through Google Scholar, general internet searches and OpenGrey (http://www.opengrey.eu/) as well as University and other data repositories.

Consider, for example, the evidence for antidepressant drugs, which are widely prescribed throughout the world. A review by Turner et al. [31] found that of 74 clinical trials of antidepressants registered with the US Food and Drug Administration, 38 had positive results, of which all but 1 was published, but 22 of the 36 trials showing no improvement were never published. Furthermore, 11 of the 14 studies with negative findings presented positive conclusions. Consequently, 94% of the trials showed that antidepressants are effective. Therefore, a systematic review that is confined to published papers might perpetuate a serious problem of bias.

Despite empirical evidence of various types of publication bias [32], reviewers rarely look beyond published data, partly due to limited time and resources but also maybe because of the legitimate concern regarding the use of non-peer reviewed data. Various tests have been devised to investigate publication bias. Most commonly used is the funnel plot, which shows each study effect size on the x-axis plotted against a measure of study size or the precision of the estimate (such as standard error) on the y-axis. When the pooled effect estimate is added to the plot, in the form of a vertical line, you would expect the studies to be approximately symmetrical around this line; remembering that this line is a summary of all of the studies. Asymmetry may be a cause for concern.

The name 'funnel plot' comes from the fact that because the y-axis shows the precision of the estimate; therefore large studies having more precise results should cluster together at the top, with these becoming more spread out as the precision falls towards the bottom, forming a triangular or inverted funnel shape. Also on the plot, there are usually lines showing the 95% confidence interval around the fixed-effects estimate, in which studies would be expected to lie in the absence of bias and heterogeneity. However, there are many reasons why you may see asymmetry in a funnel plot other than publication bias. For example, funnel plots may actually be showing small study effects, whereby smaller studies in the review really do have different results than larger studies because of the increased sampling error associated with smaller sample sizes [33]. The funnel plot associated with the forest plot above is shown in Fig. 7.3.

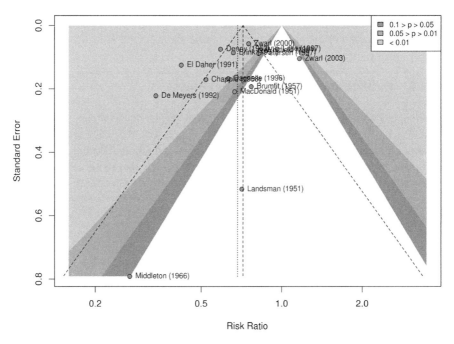

Fig. 7.3 Funnel plot of antibiotics versus placebo for treatment of sore throat (outcome: sore throat on day 3)

Although visual interpretation is useful, asymmetry in funnel pots may not always be obvious. Statistical tests for this include nonparametric rank correlation tests [34] and the regression tests for funnel plot asymmetry [35]. In the Egger test, the standard normal deviate (the effect size divided by its standard error) is regressed against the measure of precision (the inverse of the standard error), while the Begg test uses an adjusted rank correlation test between effect size and variance. The latter is nonparametric and so makes fewer assumptions about the data, but it also has more limited power to detect a statistically significant effect.

In the funnel plot above, produced by the R package *meta* [28], there certainly seems to be an area of asymmetry towards the bottom which could be indicative of publication bias. The linear regression test of funnel plot asymmetry actually shows that this asymmetry is not statistically significant, having a p-value of 0.196. As this is above the threshold of 0.05, the data *are* consistent with the null hypothesis of no asymmetry, and there is no reason to reject it in favour of the alternative hypothesis of asymmetry. However, we may still be interested in investigating the effect of this further. For this we can do a trim and fill analysis to see what effect any asymmetry may be having.

7.15 Trim and Fill

The trim and fill procedure is designed not only to detect publication bias but also to adjust for it. It consists of a number of steps:

1. Draw a funnel plot with the pooled effect size, as normal.
2. Remove (or trim) the outlying studies; there are different ways of doing this the details of which we need not go into here, but this will leave an approximately symmetrical set of studies.
3. Recalculate the pooled effect size on the remaining symmetrical studies.
4. Repeat step 2, removing any outlying studies using the new pooled effect size. Keep removing and recalculating the pooled effect size until there are no outlying studies to remove.
5. 'Fill' the funnel plot by imputing values that are symmetric to the trimmed studies.
6. Recalculate the pooled effect size using the augmented (filled) dataset.

Steps 3 and 4 may need to be repeated a number of times, until no more studies are trimmed [36]. We call this sort of process an iterative one, because it takes place a number of times and each time it 'improves' the result. In Chap. 3 on searching we said that this can also be an iterative process.

We end up with a funnel plot and result which takes account of potential missing studies, it being based on the now symmetrical filled plot. This effect size and confidence interval that you get from this procedure should not be presented as 'the result' because it is using studies that don't actually exist, but it does answer the question 'What is our best estimate of the unbiased effect size?' [37, p. 286]. This process applied to the analysis here gives a risk ratio of 0.77 with a confidence interval of

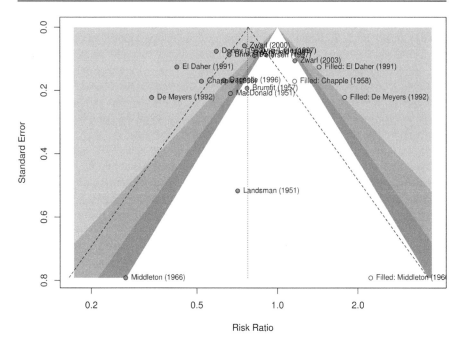

Fig. 7.4 'Trimmed and filled' funnel plot of antibiotics versus placebo for treatment of sore throat (outcome: sore throat on day 3)

0.66 to 0.91, compared to the original 0.68 (0.59–0.79); this is shown in Fig. 7.4. This suggests that the published studies might be overestimating the effect of antibiotics on reducing sore throats.

7.16   The 'File Drawer'

The 'file drawer problem', term coined by psychologist Robert Rosenthal, occurs when studies have been completed but not reported and so are stored out of sight (literally in the 'file drawer'). Had this been published today, Rosenthal might have referred to the 'hard drive/server problem'. According Rosenthal [38], 'the extreme view of the file drawer problem is that journals are filled with the 5% of the studies that show Type I errors, while the file drawers are filled with the 95% of the studies that show non-significant results'. The fail-safe number [20] is how many studies with null results would be needed to add to the pooled effect estimate to increase the level of statistical significance to a p-value of 0.05 and thus make a statistically significant result non-significant.

7.17   Sensitivity Analysis

Because undertaking a systematic review calls for a large number of decisions, we must always be cognisant of the effect of each of these on the results. Although we hope that most will be based on a clear logical process, the reality is that some will either be fairly arbitrary or the effects of our decisions not really clear. In such cases sensitivity analyses may be helpful. A sensitivity analyses is when you repeat the analysis but make alternative or different decisions to those that you actually did make [21] allowing you to get an idea of the robustness of any results to these different choices. This can be very helpful where the effect of making different decisions are not clear, for example, restricting studies to a particular geographic or clinical area, or setting some minimum methodological criteria for inclusion. Almost any decision that you make along the way can be subject to a sensitivity analysis; do it one way, and then repeat the analysis making the alternative or a different decision. One example given in the Cochrane manual we disagree with however, which is that of 'Should fixed-effect or random-effects methods be used for the analysis?' This we feel is a more fundamental issue that should be prespecified according to the nature of the desired inference.

7.18   Problems of Meta-analysis

7.18.1 Missing Data

Sometimes the data needed for a meta-analysis are not provided in papers. Remember that for mean differences, you ideally need the means of the two groups, their standard deviations and the number in each group. If any of these are not reported, you could contact the corresponding author of the paper, but be prepared for a tardy response if you get one at all.

It is also possible compute the standardised mean difference from a variety of different types of data, including raw results but also p-values. If the paper merely reports that there was no statistically significant result, you could conservatively set the standardised mean difference at 0. Similarly, if a p-value of <0.05 is given rather than the exact value, the p-value could be set at 0.04 and the standardised mean difference calculated accordingly. If means but no standard deviations are reported, it may be possible to obtain these from similar studies. There are also methods of estimating a mean and standard deviation from medians and ranges or interquartile ranges [39]. Finally for the very brave, you may hear people talking about imputation. We will not discuss this further here, but if you are interested, there is a good paper on the subject [40]. Imputation involves using the data that you do have across studies to try and estimate what the missing data might be. None of these are in any way ideal though, and by using them you run the risk of your reviewer or marker questioning your decision.

In compensating for missing data, two important principles should be applied. First, estimation based on conservative assumptions is better than excluding a study, which could cause a positive bias in findings [41]. Secondly, transparency: whatever you have done, report it clearly. You could also try undertaking a sensitivity analysis as described above, by repeating the analysis with and without the imputed or calculated data.

7.18.2 Independence of Data

An assumption of most meta-analytic models, as in statistical analysis generally, is that the data used are independent, that is, the result in one study or participant should not predict that in another. Sometimes this assumption does not hold. For example, in a study comparing a treatment that is given in clinic A with usual care in clinic B, the participants are not really independent of each other because participants are split into treatment group by clinic. This means that any difference between treatments may be due to differences between the clinics as well as because of the treatment being tested. Unwittingly, the researchers might be measuring how well the clinic staff perform rather than the treatment of interest. So independence is important for primary research, but it is also vital for meta-analysis, and there are a number of circumstances under which this independence assumption is violated.

7.18.3 Duplicate Publication

Duplicate publication is a problem whereby studies or patient data are analysed more than once in a meta-analysis as if they were different people and independent of each other. This leads to two problems, the lack of independence and that some participants are being counted twice. Sometimes it is not obvious that this has occurred, for example, studies of the same patients may have different authors or be published in different languages, or the authors have not indicated that the data have previously been published. Although the extent of duplicate publication is not known, its impact has been demonstrated in an analysis of studies comparing ondansetron with placebo for postoperative nausea and vomiting. The authors found that 17% of reported RCTs and 28% of patient data were duplicated, leading to an overestimate of the efficacy of ondansetron by 23% due to studies reporting greater efficacy being more likely to be duplicated [42].

This is an extreme example, but there are many other possible causes of data dependence in reviews, some of which are not necessarily obvious.

7.18.4 Studies That Are Linked

Sometimes you might think that studies are linked in some way, for example, if they are undertaken in the same country or hospital, for example. You might ask yourself are multiple studies conducted by a particular research group or in a particular area or country independent of each other? The patients may be different, but the effect of the common factor might influence the result. In this case you should really take account of the lack of independence which can be done by using a multi-level approach which is discussed further in a paper by Assink and Wibbelink [43].

7.18.5 More Than One Effect Size

Perhaps a more common problem is where you have an outcome that is measured using one effect size in most studies, but in one or two studies, it is measured using two effect sizes.

For example, you may be interested in an educational intervention for patients with asthma, and you have a number of studies comparing education to normal care but one study using two different types of education compared to normal care, both of which you wish to include. Just including them both as separate lines in your meta-analysis would present two problems: firstly it would lead to that study being over-weighted, and secondly it would be treating the patients in each line as being independent, which they are not as they would be using the same control group [44]. If they were not using the same control, for example, if males and females were tested using one intervention, you can simply average the two effect sizes; but if they are it is more complex because you have to take the dependence into account.

Solutions to this are to compute aggregated effect sizes; there is a function within the MAd R package [45] by the name of agg; the documentation explains 'This function will simultaneously aggregate all within-study effect sizes while taking into account the correlations among the within-study outcomes. The default correlation between outcome measures is set at 0.50, and can be adjusted as needed. An aggregate effect size and its variance is computed for each study'. The problem with this solution is that you almost certainly will not know the correlation between dependent outcomes, so you will need to use the default of 0.5 or some other value or range of values. The other approaches that you can take are to simply choose one of the interventions and remove the other, although this would lead to a loss of information, or to use a method known as robust meta-analysis which in implemented in R by a package known as robumeta [46]. This can actually fit any model as it is not affected by the type of dependence. A summary of these techniques is shown in Table 7.5 [47].

Table 7.5 Methods for managing dependencies in data

	Traditional meta-analysis	Hierarchical meta-analysis	Correlated outcomes meta-analysis
Level 1	Primary study participants		
Level 2	Provide one effect size per study	Provide effect sizes in multiple studies	Provide multiple effect sizes
Level 3		That are nested within clusters	That are nested within studies
Solutions	Traditional meta-analytic methods	Ignore clustering *or* multi-level analysis *or* robust meta-analysis	Aggregate effect sizes using known or assumed correlation *or* robust meta-analysis

7.19   Criticisms of Meta-analysis

Although meta-analysis is a powerful technique, as with all research methods it must be used with care. A common criticism is its use of 'apples and oranges'; that is studies are included that are superficially similar but actually different. Both apples and organges are fruit, but they are quite different. Heterogeneity statistics will assess differences between study results but not clinical or methodological differences. While forest plots are visually useful, they are devoid of contextual information and consequently may be misleading. For example, a meta-analysis of antibiotics for treatment of urinary tract infections is meaningless without knowing the type of infection and type of antibiotic used in each study. You don't know by looking at the forest plot in Fig. 7.2 what antibiotics the patients had, how long for, or what else might have been wrong with them. As Eysenck [48] warned 'The computer avoids the bias of the subjective approach but simply adds together the biases of the authors of the original reports - which may or may not balance out' (p. 789).

Although these criticisms have some validity, the transparency of meta-analysis is its strength. One may ask 'if not a meta-analysis, what else?' At the very least, forest plots are a powerful way of showing the results of studies, while meta-analyses should at least be transparent. Furthermore, as shown in Chap. 9, recommendations from reviews using meta-analysis may take account of heterogeneity through use of the GRADE tool [49].

7.20   If Not Meta-analysis Then What?: Narrative Reviews

If you are not going to do a meta-analysis, you need to find some other way of making sense of the data that you have. Although there is no one way of doing this, many of the principles that we have discussed in this chapter will be of use. Most importantly you will need to find a way of synthesising the studies, that is, collating and combining them before finding a way of summarising the findings [50]. It is this synthesis that differentiates a simple collection of studies from a systematic review, the 'how do you make sense of this as a body of evidence?' question. With a meta-analysis some of this is done for you, leaving you to explain and interpret the results; if you are not doing a meta-analysis, you need to find a way of doing it. At this point it may be worth just reminding those who are reading this because you are doing a course that culminates in undertaking a review; the preceding bits are generally pass/fail; you either do them right or you do not. This bit is where you can usually get the big marks, so think carefully about the method of synthesis. In their typology of reviews, Grant and Booth [51] refer to a systematic review without a meta-analysis being 'typically narrative with tabular accompaniment', with analysis that consists of:

- What is known and recommendations for practice
- What remains unknown, uncertainty around findings and recommendations for future research (p. 95)

Table 7.6   Example of data extraction table for a narrative review

Reference	Experimental result	Control result	Difference	Statistical significance	Clinical significance
Sherman et al. [4]	Mean 0.44 (SD 0.13)	Mean 0.34 (SD 0.13)	Cohen's d 0.75 CI (0.22, 1.27)	$t(58) = 2.90$ $p < 0.01$	This is for your judgement about the significance of the results

Although there are narrative methodologies, it has recently been noted that 'despite its frequent use, development of NS [narrative synthesis] methods has been scant', and that narrative syntheses often lack transparency [52, p. 8].

The most straightforward way of doing this would be to produce a table, which should contain a minimum of the study name, summary statistic, confidence interval and exact p-value if provided. Think of the data that is in each line of a forest plot, and you will get an idea as to what is needed. An example is shown in Table 7.6 below showing the data from Sherman et al. [4]. You may not want to put the clinical significance in the table like this, but it is there to remind you to make sure that you separate statistical from clinical significance. You should still consider all of the issues that we have previously discussed, such as heterogeneity, but you will not have numeric values for these.

If you are doing a table, quite a good tip for formatting is use a spreadsheet, and then use the 'format as table' menu to turn it into a table. Also balance the need to get sufficient information in with not making your table too large; it is often better to split it into two then have too much.

This brings us onto the second possibility, which is a forest plot without a meta-analysis. Within the R there are a number of packages which will draw forest plots without doing a meta-analysis, and you could probably construct one fairly easily using a drawing package as well. Because forest plots contain a lot of information and are fairly intuitive, this would be a good approach. An example of this approach was in a review looking at the effects of contact isolation on patients. We found sufficient data to pool studies looking at depression and anxiety; but for other outcomes there were not studies with the same outcomes for this to make sense, so we put these into a forest plot to present them, but we did not pool them [53].

Another idea is to use the exploratory data analysis (EDA) approach popularised by Tukey [54]. The basic goal of EDA is to seek patterns in the data in a manner analogous to detective work, that is, to answer the question 'what is going on here in these data?' It makes particular use of graphical techniques to illustrate the data, so a forest plot and other plots that one can do using meta-analysis software fit this approach; and rather than simply looking to test a hypothesis, it embraces a more iterative approach of analysis and model respecification [55]. Tukey's original book is still available, and although the graphical examples are very dated, the book predating modern graphical techniques, much of his approach can be seen in the work of today's data analysts, who look for patterns in data and produce elegant graphics.

Many of these ideas are drawn together in a formal methodology for narrative reviews by Popay et al. [56] who describe a four stage approach:

1. Develop a theory of how the intervention works, why and for whom. This is done to inform the review question and what types of studies should be included. It is also important at this stage to consider how widely applicable the results are likely to be.
2. Develop a preliminary synthesis of findings of included studies. This is done to organise the results and to look for patterns across the studies. It can be done using a variety of techniques such as textual description, clustering or grouping studies, standardising results to make them comparable, looking for common or distinct themes and content analysis.
3. Explore relationships in the data. This is done to allow consideration of factors that might explain the results. It can be done using graphical techniques such as forest and funnel plots, idea or concept mapping or textual approaches such as triangulation of method, concept or investigator, case descriptions or reciprocal and refutational translation. Here you can be really creative in how you explore the data!
4. Assess the robustness of the synthesis. This is done to provide an assessment of the strength of the evidence for the conclusions drawn and their wider generalisability. This may use the formal methods as we have already discussed or be a more reflective process.

These ideas are discussed in more detail throughout this book, for example, you may find some of the techniques associated with qualitative and mixed-methods reviews useful; and methods to assess the robustness of the synthesis are discussed later in Chap. 9.

In drawing conclusions from study results, it would be inappropriate to use a simple vote count (e.g. 'three studies were positive, two studies showed no difference, therefore the treatment works'). A nuanced conclusion will take account of studies that deserve a higher weighting than others, for example, if they have large sample sizes or narrow confidence intervals and you need to get some idea of the strength of the effect, does it work a bit better or a lot better? If the studies are small, you also run the risk of simply combining Type II errors if you are using p-values or even confidence intervals as your method of deciding if an intervention works, as both are affected by sample size. Finally you must remember that statistical significance does not equal clinical significance, and making your judgement about the efficacy of a treatment simply on p-values is not a good idea.

7.21 Software

There is a range of software which you can use to undertake a meta-analysis. These include **Cochrane Review Manager** (often referred to as RevMan) produced by the Cochrane which has the advantage of being designed for producing Cochrane Reviews and has good interactivity with other programmes such as GRADEPro. You can find *RevMan* here: https://community.cochrane.org/help/tools-and-software/revman-5.

The examples in this book have been undertaken using an R package known as *meta*: https://CRAN.R-project.org/package=meta.

Another R package for undertaking meta-analysis is ***metafor***: https://CRAN.R-project.org/package=metafor.

OpenMEE has a spreadsheet like interface: http://www.cebm.brown.edu/openmee/.

7.22 Conclusion

Meta-analysis is a widely used method of pooling quantitative data, as you can readily find in Cochrane Reviews and other evaluations of evidence. If you are doing meta-analysis, you will need to calculate the summary pooled effect estimate, the measure of variability or uncertainty, and the statistical significance (p-value). You will also need to decide whether to use a fixed-effects or random-effects model. You will be concerned with heterogeneity, and perhaps you should also assess the likelihood of publication bias. If you are unable to undertake a meta-analysis, you can use narrative techniques. Most importantly you will also need to decide on the clinical significance of the results. Whatever you do, ensure it is transparent and logical.

References

1. McKenzie JE, Brennan SE, Ryan RE, Thomson HJ, Johnston RV (2019) Chapter 9: Summarizing study characteristics and preparing for synthesis. In: Higgins JPT, Thomas J, Chandler J, Cumpston M, Li T, Page MJ, Welch VA (eds). Cochrane Handbook for Systematic Reviews of Interventions version 6.0 (updated July 2019), Cochrane. https://www.training.cochrane.org/handbook
2. Fisher RA (1948) Statistical methods for research workers, 10th edn. Oliver and Boyd, Edinburgh
3. Ranganathan P, Pramesh C, Aggarwal R (2016) Common pitfalls in statistical analysis: intention-to-treat versus per-protocol analysis. Perspect Clin Res 7:144. https://doi.org/10.4103/2229-3485.184823
4. Sherman SM, Buckley TP, Baena E, Ryan L (2016) Caffeine enhances memory performance in young adults during their non-optimal time of day. Front Psychol 7:1764. https://doi.org/10.3389/fpsyg.2016.01764
5. Fisher RA (1922) On the mathematical foundations of theoretical statistics. Phil Trans R Soc Lond A 222:309–368. https://doi.org/10.1098/rsta.1922.0009
6. Wasserstein RL, Lazar NA (2016) The ASA statement on p-values: context, process, and purpose. Am Stat 70:129–133. https://doi.org/10.1080/00031305.2016.1154108
7. Lang TA, Altman DG (2015) Basic statistical reporting for articles published in biomedical journals: the "Statistical Analyses and Methods in the Published Literature" or the SAMPL guidelines. Int J Nurs Stud 52:5–9. https://doi.org/10.1016/j.ijnurstu.2014.09.006
8. Carver R (1978) The case against statistical significance testing. Harv Educ Rev 48:378–399. https://doi.org/10.17763/haer.48.3.t490261645281841
9. Briggs M (2012) Why do statisticians answer silly questions that no one ever asks? Significance 9:30–31. https://doi.org/10.1111/j.1740-9713.2012.00542.x
10. Altman DG, Bland JM (2005) Standard deviations and standard errors. BMJ 331:903. https://doi.org/10.1136/bmj.331.7521.903

11. Glass GV (1976) Primary, secondary, and meta-analysis of research. Educ Res 5:3–8. https://doi.org/10.3102/0013189X005010003
12. Lau J, Antman EM, Jimenez-Silva J et al (1992) Cumulative meta-analysis of therapeutic trials for myocardial infarction. N Engl J Med 327:248–254. https://doi.org/10.1056/NEJM199207233270406
13. Peng C-YJ, Chen L-T (2014) Beyond Cohen's d: alternative effect size measures for between-subject designs. J Exp Educ 82:22–50. https://doi.org/10.1080/00220973.2012.745471
14. R Core Team (2020) R. A language and environment for statistical computing. R Foundation for Statistical Computing, Vienna, Austria. https://www.R-project.org/
15. Viechtbauer W (2010) Conducting meta-analyses in R with the metafor package. J Stat Softw 36(3):1–48. https://www.jstatsoft.org/v36/i03/
16. Del Re AC (2013) compute.es: Compute effect sizes R package. https://cran.r-project.org/package=compute.es
17. Cohen J (1988) Statistical power analysis for the behavioral sciences, 2nd edn. L. Erlbaum Associates, Hillsdale, NJ
18. Sawilowsky SS (2009) New effect size rules of thumb. J Mod Appl Stat Meth 8:597–599. https://doi.org/10.22237/jmasm/1257035100
19. Hedges LV, Olkin I (1980) Vote-counting methods in research synthesis. Psychol Bull 88:359–369. https://doi.org/10.1037/0033-2909.88.2.359
20. Viechtbauer W (2010) Conducting meta-analyses in R with the metafor package. J Stat Soft 36:1–48. https://doi.org/10.18637/jss.v036.i03
21. Deeks JJ, Higgins JPT, Altman DG (2019) Chapter 10: Analysing data and undertaking meta-analyses. In: Higgins JPT, Thomas J, Chandler J et al (eds) Cochrane handbook for systematic reviews of interventions version 6.0 (updated July 2019). Cochrane, London
22. Higgins JP, Thompson SG, Deeks JJ, Altman DG (2003) Measuring inconsistency in meta-analyses. BMJ (Clinical research ed.) 327(7414):557–560. https://doi.org/10.1136/bmj.327.7414.557
23. IntHout J, Ioannidis JPA, Rovers MM, Goeman JJ (2016) Plea for routinely presenting prediction intervals in meta-analysis. BMJ Open 6:e010247. https://doi.org/10.1136/bmjopen-2015-010247
24. Baker WL, White CM, Cappelleri JC et al (2009) Understanding heterogeneity in meta-analysis: the role of meta-regression. Int J Clin Pract 63:1426–1434. https://doi.org/10.1111/j.1742-1241.2009.02168.x
25. Riley RD, Lambert PC, Abo-Zaid G (2010) Meta-analysis of individual participant data: rationale, conduct, and reporting. BMJ 340:c221–c221. https://doi.org/10.1136/bmj.c221
26. Lewis S, Clarke M (2001) Forest plots: trying to see the wood and the trees. BMJ 322:1479–1480. https://doi.org/10.1136/bmj.322.7300.1479
27. Spinks A, Glasziou PP, Del Mar CB (2013) Antibiotics for sore throat. Cochrane Database Syst Rev. https://doi.org/10.1002/14651858.CD000023.pub4
28. Balduzzi S, Rücker G, Schwarzer G (2019) How to perform a meta-analysis with R: a practical tutorial. Evid Based Ment Health 22:153–160. https://doi.org/10.1136/ebmental-2019-300117
29. Brink WRR, Denny FW, Wannamaker LW (1951) Effect of penicillin and aureomycin on the natural course of streptococcal tonsillitis and pharyngitis. Am J Med 10:300–308.
30. Dickersin K, Min Y-I (1993) Publication bias: the problem that won't go away. Ann N Y Acad Sci 703:135–148. https://doi.org/10.1111/j.1749-6632.1993.tb26343.x
31. Turner EH, Matthews AM, Linardatos E et al (2008) Selective publication of antidepressant trials and its influence on apparent efficacy. N Engl J Med 358:252–260. https://doi.org/10.1056/NEJMsa065779
32. Hopewell S, Loudon K, Clarke MJ et al (2009) Publication bias in clinical trials due to statistical significance or direction of trial results. Cochrane Database Syst Rev. https://doi.org/10.1002/14651858.MR000006.pub3
33. Schwarzer G, Carpenter JR, Rücker G (2015) Meta-analysis with R. Springer International Publishing, Cham
34. Begg CB, Mazumdar M (1994) Operating characteristics of a rank correlation test for publication bias. Biometrics 50:1088–1101

35. Egger M, Smith GD, Schneider M, Minder C (1997) Bias in meta-analysis detected by a simple, graphical test. BMJ 315:629–634. https://doi.org/10.1136/bmj.315.7109.629

36. Duval S, Tweedie R (2000) A nonparametric "Trim and Fill" method of accounting for publication bias in meta-analysis. J Am Stat Assoc 95:89–98. https://doi.org/10.1080/01621459.2000.10473905

37. Borenstein M (ed) (2009) Introduction to meta-analysis. Wiley, Chichester

38. Rosenthal R (1979) The file drawer problem and tolerance for null results. Psychol Bull 86:638–641. https://doi.org/10.1037/0033-2909.86.3.638

39. Wan X, Wang W, Liu J, Tong T (2014) Estimating the sample mean and standard deviation from the sample size, median, range and/or interquartile range. BMC Med Res Methodol 14:135. https://doi.org/10.1186/1471-2288-14-135

40. Higgins JP, White IR, Wood AM (2008) Imputation methods for missing outcome data in meta-analysis of clinical trials. Clin Trials 5:225–239. https://doi.org/10.1177/1740774508091600

41. Hoyt WT, Del Re AC (2018) Effect size calculation in meta-analyses of psychotherapy outcome research. Psychother Res 28:379–388. https://doi.org/10.1080/10503307.2017.1405171

42. Tramèr MR, Reynolds DJM, Moore RA, McQuay HJ (1997) Impact of covert duplicate publication on meta-analysis: a case study. BMJ 315:635–640. https://doi.org/10.1136/bmj.315.7109.635

43. Assink M, Wibbelink CJM (2016) Fitting three-level meta-analytic models in R: a step-by-step tutorial. TQMP 12:154–174. https://doi.org/10.20982/tqmp.12.3.p154

44. Van den Noortgate W, López-López JA, Marín-Martínez F, Sánchez-Meca J (2013) Three-level meta-analysis of dependent effect sizes. Behav Res 45:576–594. https://doi.org/10.3758/s13428-012-0261-6

45. Del Re A, Hoyt W (2014) MAd: meta-analysis with mean differences. R package version 0.8-2. https://cran.r-project.org/package=MAd

46. Fisher Z, Tipton E, Zhipeng H (2017) robumeta: Robust variance meta-regression. R package version 2.0. https://CRANR-project.org/package=robumeta

47. Tanner-Smith EE, Tipton E, Polanin JR (2016) Handling complex meta-analytic data structures using robust variance estimates: a tutorial in R. J Dev Life Course Criminol 2:85–112. https://doi.org/10.1007/s40865-016-0026-5

48. Eysenck HJ (1994) Systematic reviews: meta-analysis and its problems. BMJ 309:789–792. https://doi.org/10.1136/bmj.309.6957.789

49. Schünemann H, Brożek J, Guyatt G, Oxman A (2013) GRADE handbook. https://gdt.gradepro.org/app/handbook/handbook.html. Accessed 6 Mar 2020

50. Centre for Reviews and Dissemination (2009) CRD's guidance for undertaking reviews in healthcare, 3rd edn. York Publ. Services, York

51. Grant MJ, Booth A (2009) A typology of reviews: an analysis of 14 review types and associated methodologies: A typology of reviews. Health Inform Libr J 26:91–108. https://doi.org/10.1111/j.1471-1842.2009.00848.x

52. Campbell M, Katikireddi SV, Sowden A, Thomson H (2019) Lack of transparency in reporting narrative synthesis of quantitative data: a methodological assessment of systematic reviews. J Clin Epidemiol 105:1–9. https://doi.org/10.1016/j.jclinepi.2018.08.019

53. Purssell E, Gould D, Chudleigh J (2020) Impact of isolation on hospitalised patients who are infectious: systematic review with meta-analysis. BMJ Open 10:e030371. https://doi.org/10.1136/bmjopen-2019-030371

54. Tukey JW (1977) Exploratory data analysis. Addison-Wesley Publ. Co., Reading, MA

55. Behrens JT (1997) Principles and procedures of exploratory data analysis. Psychol Methods 2:131–160. https://doi.org/10.1037/1082-989X.2.2.131

56. Popay J, Roberts H, Sowden A, et al (2006) Guidance on the conduct of narrative synthesis in systematic reviews. A product from the ESRC Methods Programme. https://www.researchgate.net/publication/233866356_Guidance_on_the_conduct_of_narrative_synthesis_in_systematic_reviews_A_product_from_the_ESRC_Methods_Programme

Reviewing Qualitative Studies and Metasynthesis

8

Summary Learning Points
- Qualitative reviews may be undertaken by a variety of approaches, of which metasynthesis is perhaps the most common.
- Data are typically extracted in an iterative way, moving backwards and forwards between review stages, revisiting study reports as the synthesis proceeds.
- The precise approach should be informed by the purpose of the synthetic product.
- Reviews may be primarily to produce practical knowledge or a contribution to theoretical development that engages readers at a philosophical level.

Whereas the product of quantitative research is expressed by number, there is no such brevity with qualitative research. Taking a step back from research, consider a film review in a newspaper. Alongside an image, there may be half a page of text presenting the reviewer's impression of the merits of the acting, production and storyline. This is all qualitative information, but there is usually a quantitative element too. At the end of the review is a rating. The quality of a movie may be judged by reading the reviewer's account or simply by the number of stars awarded. To satisfy the different preferences of readers, most newspapers provide both types of data in their review sections, whether for books, plays, films or music. Some readers give more prominence to the score; others prefer the descriptive detail.

If you were interested in comparing reviews of a particular film, you could start by collating the ratings in the various newspapers and periodicals. Gathering and tabulating these quantitative data are relatively straightforward, and by standardising the denominator (ratings may have different ranges), you could readily calculate a mean score (e.g. 3.2 out of 5). By contrast, dealing with the many thousands of words of the textual reviews will take you much more time. Furthermore, it is not inherently clear what you will produce from this exercise. Arguably, if you simply want to show whether the film is good or bad, you might as well just count the stars. In this chapter we assume that you want to do more than condense the findings of qualitative studies into a single statement. That is neither the purpose of qualitative research, nor a review of qualitative research.

© The Editor(s) (if applicable) and The Author(s), under exclusive license to Springer Nature Switzerland AG 2020
E. Purssell, N. McCrae, *How to Perform a Systematic Literature Review*, https://doi.org/10.1007/978-3-030-49672-2_8

103

Existentialist philosopher Martin Buber [1], in his classic treatise *I and Thou* (1923), differentiated subjective and objective ways of seeing as 'I-thou' and 'I-it'. We may treat others as a unique person (an I-thou relationship) or reduce them to a purpose (I-it). In a bureaucratic organisation, the role specification is officially more important than the character of the employee. In reality, however, workplaces are social as well as instrumental, and often an unofficial hierarchy exists [2]. At a supermarket checkout, an I-thou exchange occurs if the customer or till operator genuinely takes interest in each other, however fleetingly; more frequently the relationship is I-it, whereby the customer sees the till operator as a mere conduit to the purchase.

This relational conceptualisation is helpful in understanding the fundamental difference between qualitative and quantitative enquiry. Personal experience can be objectified by use of a standardised instrument, for example, to measure mood. However, the score is merely a proxy representation: the person does not really feel 22.5 out of 30. In healthcare and in healthcare research, both objective and subjective approaches are necessary. The practitioner applies evidence-based interventions but should also be tuned to the personal reality of the patient. The body consists of quantifiable matter, but the person is a sentient being, who has presence. Qualitative research focuses on how people see the world, acknowledging that each participant has their own version of truth on the phenomenon of interest. A systematic review of qualitative research must preserve this essence.

8.1   Reviewing Qualitative Studies

Back in the 1980s, sociologists were working on ways to integrate findings from diverse qualitative studies into a comprehensive and coherent account. The technique of metatheory was described by Ritzer [3] and Zhao [4]. A seminal text was *Meta-Ethnography: Synthesising Qualitative Studies* by educational theorists Noblit and Hare [5]. In this manual, Noblit and Hare presented the process of reciprocal translational analysis. This entails systematically comparing or concepts or themes across and within study accounts. By 'translation', Noblit and Hare did not mean converting one language to another (as the term is generally used) but a systematic comparison of meaning to generate broader explanation of a phenomenon. All social knowledge is both contextual and comparative. Reciprocal translational analysis is similar to the constant comparison technique in grounded theory [6]. It is key to meta-ethnography, which became the most common structured approach to reviewing qualitative studies in social sciences.

In the field of healthcare, it was nursing, with its predilection for qualitative research, where reviewing methodology was most keenly pursued. A provocative paper by Estabrooks et al. [7] urged qualitative researchers to stop wasting time on ad hoc original studies and to focus instead on the 'incremental business of accumulating knowledge'. Perhaps the earliest qualitative synthesis in nursing was by Jensen and Allen [8] at the University of Alberta, on the relationship between wellness and illness. The term 'metasynthesis' was first used by Stern and Harris in a review of women's self-care. Jensen and Allen [9] then presented a framework for metasynthesis, with two stages of synthesising: hermeneutic (accurately portraying individual study accounts) and dialectic (comparing and contrasting the accounts). Inspired by the work of Noblit and Hare, metasynthesis was further developed by nursing scholars Sally Thorne, Deborah Finfgeld, Cheryl Beck, Margaret Kearney, Julie Barroso and Margarete Sandelowski.

The term 'meta-analysis' (coined by Glass for analysing quantitative study results) was used by some qualitative reviewers in nursing. However, there is an important philosophical difference between analysis and synthesis. According to the *Oxford Dictionary of Philosophy* [10], analysis is to reduce a concept into its core elements, thus revealing its logical structure. Synthesis is the product of resolving the conflict between one proposition and another (thesis and antithesis). This is the dialectical process described by nineteenth-century philosopher Georg Hegel. Relating these definitions to literature reviewing, analysis examines study data or findings and discerns common themes, while synthesis integrates multiple and possibly divergent study findings to generate theory.

Although it began as a distinct approach to integrating findings from multiple qualitative studies, 'metasynthesis' has become a generic term for reviewing qualitative research [11]. However, a report for the ESRC National Centre for Research Methods by Barnett-Page and Thomas [12] described nine methods of synthesising qualitative studies: meta-narrative, critical interpretative synthesis, meta-study, meta-ethnography, grounded formal theory, thematic synthesis, textual narrative synthesis, framework synthesis and ecological triangulation. While not overlooking the value of specialised approaches, for the purpose of this chapter, we are wary of complicating the process unnecessarily (readers particularly interested in critical interpretative methods, for example, should consult relevant texts). We use metasynthesis for a systematic review that interprets rather than merely summarises the findings of qualitative studies. Such a broad definition might displease purists, but in practice we would argue that meta-ethnography, metasynthesis and other methods have considerably more similarity than difference.

8.2 Process of Metasynthesis

As an interpretative integration of interpretative study findings, metasynthesis is not just truth-seeking but also truth-making [11]. The phrase 'a whole greater than the sum of parts' should apply to the product of any systematic review, but it is particularly relevant to metasynthesis, which does not merely aggregate study findings. Unlike the procedural process of systematically reviewing RCTs or other quantitative studies, metasynthesis is both art and science [11]. It is a complex, creative endeavour not suited to the concrete thinker.

Among the challenges is the variation in methods used in the reviewed studies. Grounded theory and ethnography, for example, are based on different epistemology (a philosophical stance on how truth can be found). Basically, an ethnographer is concerned with cultural meanings, while a study applying grounded theory investigates a phenomenon for the purpose of sociological theory. These epistemological differences are important considerations for the reviewer in interpreting and integrating findings.

Another difficulty may be the sufficiency of information in a qualitative study report. Presentation of data and findings is constrained by journal word limits. Some qualitative researchers are better than others at distilling a vast set of data and interpretations into a few thousand words. The reviewer may also find a wide range in the length and depth of study reports, from a verbose tract of phenomenological analysis to a rudimentary descriptive account (perhaps as an addendum to a quantitative study).

An accessible guide to metasynthesis was presented by Walsh and Downe in the *Journal of Advanced Nursing* [13]. Closely following the ethnographic approach of Noblit and Hare [5], Walsh and Downe described two ways of seeing the original data and findings. The first is hermeneutic, which entails accurately portraying the meanings in original data. The second is dialectic: comparing and contrasting, showing similarities and differences. In ethnography, these relate to emic and etic perspectives. Hermeneutic meaning is derived from the internal (emic) data and analysis; in other words, subjective individual and collective experiences and behaviour in their context. Dialectic reasoning contrasts the emic account with other contexts, thus externalising the enquiry.

There may be much overlap in study findings but sometimes conflicting ideas and explanations. The reviewer must not impose homogeneity, but pursue a genuinely holistic synthesis: as Noblit and Hare [5] emphasised, reciprocal translation finds a common language to represent the various interpretations, but it should preserve the uniqueness of primary findings. Although a consensus may emerge, a 'tyranny of the majority' is antithetical.

Sandelowski and Barroso produced a manual for metasynthesis, which they defined as 'an interpretive integration of qualitative findings in primary research reports that are in the form of interpretive syntheses of data: either conceptual/thematic descriptions or interpretive explanations' [14, p. 199]. Their method, which emphasises trustworthiness and credibility, comprises four processes:

1. Comprehensive search
2. Appraisal of studies
3. Classification of studies
4. Synthesis of findings

There are two stages of synthesis in this model. First, findings of the studies are assembled in a metasummary. This entails extraction, separation, grouping and abstraction of findings into a set of statements. Although a numerical tally cannot convey the meaning to be derived from rich qualitative data, Sandelowski and Barroso recommended counting to show the strength of patterns and theoretical propositions. Often reviewers present percentages in a metasummary table, showing how frequently a concept appeared in the research findings. Ludvigsen and colleagues [15] explained the value of this activity:

> We found that integrating findings into metasummaries was not only a technical issue but also an iterative process whereby the research team moved towards consensus in the analysis before moving on to the final metasynthesis step. Counting helped us focus on similarities, differences, strengths, and variations in gender, number of participants, origin of countries, and methodologies.

After the metasummary is produced, metasynthesis proper can begin. Sandelowski and Barroso explained the reciprocal translation of Noblit and Hare [5] as an integrating process, combining in vivo concepts from a study with concepts imported from other studies. Metasynthesis is the ultimate stage; this is on a higher plane of abstraction, producing new concepts and theoretical propositions. The final product is not necessarily congruent: if there is tension between study findings, synthesis should show this.

As argued by Barnett-Page and Thomas [12] in their description of qualitative review methods, the approach to synthesis should be informed by the purpose of the synthetic product. A review may be primarily to produce practical knowledge or a contribution to theoretical development that engages readers at a philosophical level. Humility should be shown by the qualitative reviewer: no single theory can comprehensively or enduringly explain a phenomenon; in the humanities, knowledge is in constant flux.

8.3   Data Extraction

Qualitative data extraction is not as straightforward as in reviews of quantitative research. Often it entails moving backwards and forwards between review stages, revisiting study reports as the synthesis proceeds. Review teams (or student and supervisor) should meet regularly to consider the data and findings and reach a consensual understanding. As Noyes and colleagues [16] described in the qualitative chapter of the Cochrane handbook, whatever the method of synthesis, it is best practice to extract contextual and methodological information on each study and to report this information in Table 8.1. The reviewer should ensure that the context of original studies is preserved in the extraction process, to prevent misinterpretation. A data extraction form should comprise the following:

Reviewers may use a generic data extraction template, as developed by the National Institute for Health and Care Excellence [17] or devise a bespoke template tailored to the review topic. Another approach is to use a 'best fit' framework [18]: this entails finding an appropriate theory or conceptual model for investigating the phenomenon of interest, with evidence from the studies coded against the themes of the a priori framework. The 'PROGRESS' formulation is useful in ensuring an equitable focus [19]: place of residence, race/ethnicity/culture/language, occupation, gender/sex, religion, education, socioeconomic status and social capital.

Various electronic software packages may be used for inductive extraction from qualitative studies. Most software for the analysis of primary qualitative data, such as NVivo (QSR International, accessed 2 March 2020), may be used to code studies

Table 8.1 Data extraction for qualitative studies [16]

Data extraction field	Information to extract
Context and participants	Important elements of study context relevant to the review question, specifying the study setting, population profile, participants and intervention (if applicable)
Study design and methods used	Methodological approach, sampling, data collection, analysis and any theoretical model used to interpret or contextualise the findings

in a systematic review. If you search in Google Scholar for qualitative studies on a chosen topic and add NVivo to your search terms, you are sure to find many papers (e.g. a quick search for 'qualitative', 'social media' and 'NVivo' reaps nearly 9000 results). Just as thematic analysis is used by primary researchers to analyse their data, this can be applied to extracting data and themes in a synthesis of qualitative studies.

8.4   Examples of Metasyntheses

Qualitative research is valuable in exploring complex, abstract phenomena that defy positivist investigation. The humanistic practice and interpersonal dynamics of healthcare are not readily converted into cause-and-effect variables for experimental testing. Here are two examples of metasyntheses that examine metaphysical aspects of nursing: one reviewing studies of 'presence' and the other a review of 'hope' among family carers.

Nursing scholar Finfgeld-Connett [20] applied her own, previously published method of metasynthesis [21] in a review of presence in nursing. This was a concept much discussed in nursing literature but difficult to delineate, and theorists and researchers have conflated it with other concepts such as caring, empathy and therapeutic use of self. Included in the metasynthesis were 14 qualitative studies and 4 linguistic concept analyses. An initial coding schema was based on a formulation of antecedents, attributes and consequences. Substantive categories were developed, applying the grounded theory principle of saturation. A model was created with links between constructs. Finfgeld-Connett concluded that presence depends on the receptiveness of the patient, the willingness of the nurse and a conducive environment. Nurses who convey positive presence have personal and professional maturity, and their practice is steered by the moral principle of commitment. Rewards derived from presence encourage its future enactment.

Duggleby and colleagues [22] applied the method of Sandelowski and Barroso [14] in a review of qualitative studies of hope in family carers of persons with chronic illness. These studies produced very different findings on the hope and despair of carers. The three-stage process of synthesis was described as follows:

> Synthesis of the findings was achieved using taxonomic analysis, constant target comparison and reciprocal translation. The purpose of the taxonomic analysis was to identify significant underlying concepts and conceptual relationships. The study findings were then evaluated for similarities and differences to clarify defining and overlapping attributes of hope and discern relationships among the interpreted concepts. Reciprocal translations of the concepts were then used to integrate the metasynthesis findings.

The 14 studies included in the review by Duggleby and colleagues were of various qualitative design, including 7 grounded theory studies, 3 using phenomenology and 1 ethnography. Metasynthesis resulted in a new conceptual model, defining hope as 'transitional dynamic possibilities within uncertainty'. It is the uncertain future that leaves doors open for hopefulness, and this boosts resilience.

8.5 Ensuring Rigour

Thorne's [23] paper 'Metasynthetic Madness: What Kind of Monster Have We Created?' argued that the method has been diluted and distorted from its original purpose. Noting that application of metasynthesis in journal articles increased from 38 in 2000 to 3250 in 2015, Thorne found that many reviewers present merely a descriptive summary of findings. Thorne [24] worried that novice reviewers are being led astray:

> Increasingly, young scholars are being encouraged to formulate their literature reviews into a tightly focused and highly structured process, along the lines advocated by the Cochrane Collaboration, for which the defining feature is a predetermined searching, screening and summarizing rubric applied to answering a narrow research question.

Consequently, reviews are more aggregative than interpretative, with reviewers 'counting or tabulating qualitative research results into reports that sum up the major thematic findings extracted from each study and reduce them to the most commonly reported categorizations—which would seem to defeat the purpose'. Overly structured but shallow synthesis erodes or erases the 'texture, color, and contour that was the essence of the high quality original qualitative research product'. The goal of metasynthesis is not a single truth but 'ideas that will enlighten, enrich, elaborate, and enhance the understandings with which one approaches real-life problems in the health arena' [24].

Instead of appearing as a technical report, with little inductive enquiry, a metasynthesis should generate a unique interpretative product. Thorne [23] proposed the following quality criteria:

- Are the exclusion processes justified by the explicit aims of the review?
- Have the mechanisms for data display demonstrably furthered the analytic capacity?
- Is there evidence of critical reflection on the role played by method, theoretical framework, disciplinary orientation and local conditions in shaping the studies under consideration?
- Does the interpretation of the body of available studies reflect an understanding of the influence of chronological sequence and advances in thought within the field over time?
- Does the synthesis tell us something about the collection of studies that we would not have known without a rigorous and systematic process of cross-interrogation?

Rigour in qualitative enquiry must not be defined by the premises of quantitative research. Bergdahl [25] of Nord University in Norway criticised the emergence of meta-aggregation as a systematic method of reviewing qualitative research. As described by Lockwood and colleagues [26], meta-aggregation mimics the quantitative approach to systematic reviewing as closely as possible while acknowledging the distinctiveness of qualitative findings. However, Bergdahl argued that the aggregative method is incompatible with the 'epistemological, philosophical and ethical foundation of the qualitative research tradition'. Indeed, it was after realising the reductionist limitations of aggregating in their review of research on racial desegregation in American schools that Noblit and Hare [5] devised meta-ethnography.

A qualitative synthesis is a sophisticated endeavour. Bergdahl [25] warned reviewers not to 'turn rich descriptions into thin abstractions'. In supervising students working on dissertations, we often see qualitative findings presented as 'themes' that are actually not thematic. For example, one student who was reviewing qualitative studies on patients' experience of waiting for surgery had themes such as 'waiting time' and 'information provided'. This was simply a generalised sorting of information, descriptive rather than interpretative and subtracting from rather than adding to the knowledge generated by the studies. An interpretative approach could have produced themes such as 'stoicism', 'feeling stuck' or 'projecting anxiety on to others'. However, there is no single truth, and while some experiences may be common, the aim of metasynthesis is to make sense of all individual perspectives.

Qualitative reviewers should always remember that all studies are contextual, and each participant speaks in context.

Creativity and critical thinking are vital to metasynthesis. Meaning does not simply emerge from the original data or findings but from the theoretical application of the reviewer. Aggregation of findings may be useful as a descriptive exercise, but it does not entail interpretation or theoretical input. It is deductive and influenced by the positivist tradition of science. Metasynthesis, by contrast, embraces multiple truths in an inductive pursuit of theory.

8.6   Conclusion

Metasynthesis is necessarily art and science, and proficiency is gained not only from procedural manuals but from trial and error. The fundamental principles and practice of this method have been shown here, but the quality of synthesis depends on the creativity and theoretical intuition of the reviewer. Ultimately, a good metasynthesis produces new theory from existing studies or as Sandelowski [27] described: 'fuller knowledge'.

References

1. Buber M, Smith RG (2010) I and Thou. Martino Publishing, Mansfield Centre, CT
2. Pugh DS, Hickson DJ (2007) Writers on organizations, 6th edn. Penguin, London
3. Ritzer G (1990) Metatheorizing in sociology. Sociol Forum 5:3–15. https://doi.org/10.1007/BF01115134
4. Zhao S (1991) Metatheory, metamethod, meta-data-analysis: what, why, and how? Sociol Perspect 34:377–390. https://doi.org/10.2307/1389517

5. Noblit GW, Hare RD (1988) Meta-ethnography: synthesizing qualitative studies. Sage Publications, Newbury Park
6. Glaser BG, Strauss A (1967) The discovery of grounded theory, Aldine de Gruyter, New York
7. Estabrooks CA, Field PA, Morse JM (1994) Aggregating qualitative findings: an approach to theory development. Qual Health Res 4:503–511. https://doi.org/10.1177/104973239400400410
8. Jensen LA, Allen MN (1994) A synthesis of qualitative research on wellness-illness. Qual Health Res 4:349–369. https://doi.org/10.1177/104973239400400402
9. Jensen LA, Allen MN (1996) Meta-synthesis of qualitative findings. Qual Health Res 6:553–560. https://doi.org/10.1177/104973239600600407
10. Blackburn S (2008) The Oxford dictionary of philosophy, 2nd rev. edn. Oxford University Press, Oxford
11. Thorne S, Jensen L, Kearney MH et al (2004) Qualitative metasynthesis: reflections on methodological orientation and ideological agenda. Qual Health Res 14:1342–1365. https://doi.org/10.1177/1049732304269888
12. Barnett-Page E, Thomas J (2009) Methods for the synthesis of qualitative research: a critical review. ESRC National Centre for Research Methods, London
13. Walsh D, Downe S (2005) Meta-synthesis method for qualitative research: a literature review. J Adv Nurs 50:204–211. https://doi.org/10.1111/j.1365-2648.2005.03380.x
14. Sandelowski M, Barroso J (2007) Handbook for synthesizing qualitative research. Springer Publishing Company, New York
15. Ludvigsen MS, Hall EOC, Meyer G et al (2016) Using Sandelowski and Barroso's meta-synthesis method in advancing qualitative evidence. Qual Health Res 26:320–329. https://doi.org/10.1177/1049732315576493
16. Noyes J, Booth A, Cargo M et al (2019) Chapter 21: Qualitative evidence. In: Higgins JPT, Thomas J, Chandler J et al (eds) Cochrane handbook for systematic reviews of interventions version 6.0 (updated July 2019). Cochrane, London. https://www.training.cochrane.org/handbook
17. National Institute for Health and Care Excellence (2012) Methods for the development of NICE public health guidance. Process and Methods [PMG4], 3rd edn. NICE. https://www.nice.org.uk/process/pmg4/chapter/introduction. Accessed 6 Mar 2020
18. Carroll C, Booth A, Leaviss J, Rick J (2013) "Best fit" framework synthesis: refining the method. BMC Med Res Methodol 13:37. https://doi.org/10.1186/1471-2288-13-37
19. O'Neill J, Tabish H, Welch V et al (2014) Applying an equity lens to interventions: using PROGRESS ensures consideration of socially stratifying factors to illuminate inequities in health. J Clin Epidemiol 67:56–64. https://doi.org/10.1016/j.jclinepi.2013.08.005
20. Finfgeld-Connett D (2006) Meta-synthesis of presence in nursing. J Adv Nurs 55:708–714. https://doi.org/10.1111/j.1365-2648.2006.03961.x
21. Finfgeld DL (2003) Metasynthesis: the state of the art—so far. Qual Health Res 13:893–904. https://doi.org/10.1177/1049732303253462
22. Duggleby W, Holtslander L, Kylma J et al (2010) Metasynthesis of the hope experience of family caregivers of persons with chronic illness. Qual Health Res 20:148–158. https://doi.org/10.1177/1049732309358329
23. Thorne S (2017) Metasynthetic madness: what kind of monster have we created? Qual Health Res 27:3–12. https://doi.org/10.1177/1049732316679370
24. Thorne S (2019) On the evolving world of what constitutes qualitative synthesis. Qual Health Res 29:3–6. https://doi.org/10.1177/1049732318813903
25. Bergdahl E (2019) Is meta-synthesis turning rich descriptions into thin reductions? A criticism of meta-aggregation as a form of qualitative synthesis. Nurs Inq 26:e12273. https://doi.org/10.1111/nin.12273
26. Lockwood C, Munn Z, Porritt K (2015) Qualitative research synthesis: methodological guidance for systematic reviewers utilizing meta-aggregation. Int J Evid Based Healthc 13:179–187. https://doi.org/10.1097/XEB.0000000000000062
27. Sandelowski M (1993) Rigor or rigor mortis: the problem of rigor in qualitative research revisited. Adv Nurs Sci 16:1–8. https://doi.org/10.1097/00012272-199312000-00002

Reviewing Qualitative and Quantitative Studies and Mixed-Method Reviews

9

Summary Learning Points
- Combining quantitative and qualitative research in a systematic review may allow for valuable insights but can be complicated.
- It is important to use a recognised methodology to help manage this complexity.
- The most common approach is the segregated review, where qualitative and quantitative findings are analysed separately, before synthesising them.
- Integrated approaches require that study findings are transformed in some way to make them directly comparable. Quantitative results may be converted to qualitative findings or vice versa.
- Contingent approaches allow one group of studies to inform the other in a sequential way.
- Findings may be convergent, divergent or similar. Each is important.

In the healthcare setting, there is general acceptance that patients' perspectives should be valued alongside generalised knowledge from scientific testing. In a debrief after an adverse incident on a hospital ward, two questions are asked of the doctors and nurses involved. First, what happened? This requires factual information, which may be corroborated. Second, how did you feel? This question seeks a subjective view but a feeling such as distress is as real as the detail of events. A reciprocal account is produced, using both types of testimony. A report based only on factual detail will be incomplete.

Indeed, inclusion of the subjective experience of recipients of care is strongly recommended by major research funding bodies and by the GRADE approach to making recommendations from a systematic review (see Chap. 9). Therefore, a reviewer may be inclined to encompass qualitative and quantitative studies on the chosen topic. The term 'mixed-method review' has an intuitive appeal, to many would-be reviewers, promising as it does to relieve the stress of deciding if the search should concentrate upon quantitative or qualitative research. However, we advise proceeding with caution, because major philosophical and practical challenges await the ecumenical novice. Upon commencing the review, the full enormity of the task will become clear, and we would advise great caution about taking this on. Although

E. Purssell, N. McCrae, *How to Perform a Systematic Literature Review*, https://doi.org/10.1007/978-3-030-49672-2_9

the quantitative/qualitative divide is much less than it used to be, most researchers will tend towards one or the other, and there are still very fundamental differences that make aggregating them difficult.

Postmodern philosopher Midgley [1] rejected the separation of scientific truth from moral concerns, criticising reductionism and urging a pluralistic approach to knowledge. In healthcare, the need for different perspectives has been advanced by the likes of Greenhalgh [2], and mixing of quantitative and qualitative paradigms is increasingly common in research on treatments and services. Mixed-method research is based on the premise that both objective and subjective data are valid sources of knowledge.

The difference between subjective and objective realities is akin to the dualism of structure and agency. Structure does not necessarily mean physical surroundings but social forces that predict how people will behave. Norms, for example, are abstract but very real in governing our behaviour. By contrast, agency is the individual exercise of free will. For example, consider how you decided what clothes to wear today. Structure sets standards of acceptability, but you will probably think that the choice was entirely yours.

Quantitative methods may be used to measure cause-and-effect relationships or to estimate the frequency of a condition, typically from a sample that represents a population producing generalisable results. The status of this evidence is rarely deterministic but probabilistic. This is a structural truth: statistically, people are more or less likely to get a disease or to recover with a tested treatment if certain predictive factors apply. Qualitative methods are in the domain of agency, which is where we find phenomenal truth. Each human being has unique experiences and perspectives, and participants in a qualitative study represent nobody but themselves.

This contrast in outlook shows that there are fundamental philosophical challenges in mixed-method research. One paradigm posits external reality, while the other believes that there are as many truths as there are people. In the ontology of realism, objective scientific investigation is the means to discover facts, causal relationships and universal laws. Since the postmodern turn in social sciences in the 1960s, with its critique of scientific hegemony, the ontology of idealism has come to the fore. Social scientists emphasise the social construction of knowledge, with behaviour dependent on meanings generated in a community or wider culture. From a relativist stance, one group may have a different truth to that believed by another group: there is no absolute truth. As Wootton [3] suggested, both sides of the realism/idealism divide should be humble:

> Realists are wrong to deny any social construction in science. Relativists are wrong to assert that science is only a social construct.

Some research methodologists argue that mixing the paradigms is untenable (e.g. [4]), but others reject such absolutism as an obstacle to the advance of science. According to social scientist Hammersley [5], the differences have been overstated, as both quantitative and qualitative methods are systematic, empirical pursuits of knowledge. The research cycle moves from observations to inferences through inductive logic and from hypotheses to observations through deductive reasoning: wherever it starts, all research is on this cycle of ideas and data (Tashakkori and Teddlie [6]).

9.1 Mixed-Method Studies

As a first principle of mixed-method research, there should be a single overarching research question, which the methods are answering in different ways. However, synthesising the findings from different methods is challenging. What is their relative importance? Take these two examples of study findings:

- A drug is highly effective in alleviating symptoms but has some troubling side effects.
- A new service in primary care is successful in reducing hospital admissions but raises the burden on family carers.

The first study could be an experimental trial, with multiple outcomes measured quantitatively, including side effects. A qualitative component may be included to explore patients' experiences related to the treatment, but typically this will be of supplementary rather than equal status to the statistical results. The second study is a service evaluation and will be more elaborate in design. As recommended by research funding bodies such as the Medical Research Council, complex interventions should be evaluated with attention to process as well as outcomes. Therefore, qualitative enquiry is needed to explain *how* things happen, as well as counting *how much* something happened. Qualitative data are considerably more valued in the latter type of study.

Ideally, a mixed-method study should be published intact, rather than being split into qualitative and quantitative reports. If the study has answered a question from different angles, the benefits of triangulation may be lost. Partly due to journal requirements, qualitative findings are often presented in a different place from the quantitative report. The reviewer who is interested in studies that investigate process and outcome should be aware that mixed-method research is not always published intact. Authors will normally link their work in their papers, so that the study can be reassembled for review purposes.

9.2 Approaching a Mixed-Method Review

Whatever the research question, making sense of a combination of qualitative and quantitative findings is challenging. This is particularly difficult for a reviewer of evidence deriving from statistical and interpretative studies.

Three general approaches may be made to the material of a mixed-method review [7]:

- *Segregated*: The most common approach is to analyse qualitative and quantitative findings separately, before synthesising them. A segregated approach maintains the methodological logic of each paradigm. Comparison of the two sets of findings may incline towards confirmation or refutation. Often found is partial complementarity, whereby the findings are not fully concordant but have meaningful overlap.
- *Integrated*: In an integrated approach, study findings are transformed in some way to make them directly comparable. Quantitative results may be converted to qualitative findings, or vice versa.
- *Contingent*: In a contingent approach, analysis of a subset of studies is used to inform analysis of the next subset. Studies are grouped not by method but by the question that they answered.

9.3   Segregation and Synthesis

An authoritative source of methodological guidance and tools for mixed-method research is the Joanna Briggs Institute. An international collaboration of healthcare researchers and clinicians, this organisation was founded in 1996 in the name of the first matron of the Royal Adelaide Hospital in Australia, and it established a base at the University of Adelaide. In 2005, the Joanna Briggs Institute Model for Evidence-Based Healthcare was introduced. This developmental framework for evidence-based practice showed how research evidence relates to theory and practice. It was recently updated with an emphasis on utilisation [8]. Evidence-based healthcare, according to the Joanna Briggs Institute model, must be feasible, appropriate, meaningful and effective. In the complex, contextual environment of healthcare, evidence is pluralistic, including not only research findings but also practitioners' expertise and patients' experience. The model comprises four activities:

- Evidence generation
- Evidence synthesis
- Evidence transfer
- Evidence utilisation (renamed 'implementation' in revised version)

Most relevant here is evidence synthesis, which is predominantly achieved by systematic reviewing. The Joanna Briggs Institute [9] emphasises the dual need for evidence on process and outcomes. Its favoured approach is segregated analysis of quantitative and qualitative findings. For quantitative studies, this entails meta-analysis (as discussed in Chap. 6), which combines the results of studies into a pooled estimate with confidence interval and assessment of statistical heterogeneity. For qualitative studies, the Joanna Briggs Institute uses the term 'meta-aggregation', which has three stages:

1. *Extracting findings from papers*: Qualitative study findings are the author's interpretation of the data, in the writing style of the author, illustrated by quotes or observations. Credibility may be judged as follows:
   - Unequivocal: the finding is presented beyond reasonable doubt.
   - Credible: the finding is plausible but has insufficient explanation or illustration.
   - Unsupported: the finding is not supported by the data and therefore should not be included in synthesis.
2. *Aggregate similar findings into categories*: Categories are comprised of two or more similar findings. A category description conveys the meaning of the findings within that category.
3. *Group categories into synthesised findings*: Two or more categories are grouped into synthesised findings, with explanatory notes. Synthesised findings should be shaped into explicit statements that guide practice or policy, rather than implicit or vague contributions to theory.

Quantitative data should be analysed using a random effects meta-analysis. If this is not possible, study results should be presented in a tabular summary showing the intervention, participants and other contextual information and results with measures of dispersion (confidence intervals or standard deviations). For more information on this, see Chap. 6.

The Joanna Briggs Institute method also embraces economic analysis. Such evidence should be summarised numerically and/or in narrative form. Economics is satirised as the 'dismal science', and arguably health economics is the most dismal of all! Costs are very difficult to calculate in the context of family support and complex health and social care systems, with wide variation between countries. Nonetheless, economic analysis is increasingly demanded by research funding bodies, as policy-makers and healthcare providers want to know not only whether a treatment works but also its expense relative to existing treatment.

9.4 Converting Findings from One Paradigm to Another

Synthesis of the separately aggregated qualitative and quantitative findings may be facilitated by making them directly comparable. It is possible to transform quantitative results to a verbal form that can be interpreted rather than statistically analysed. According to the Joanna Briggs Institute [9], 'codifying quantitative data is less error-prone than attributing numerical values to qualitative data'. The coded quantitative results and qualitative findings are analysed separately and then combined for an overall synthesis.

Similarly, qualitative findings may be quantified, although it is trickier to represent words by number. Meta-analysis of the converted qualitative findings would not be possible because this needs not only an estimate of effect but also measures of dispersion (confidence interval or standard deviation). Therefore, aggregation would comprise two sets of analyses: quantified qualitative findings and meta-analysed quantitative results.

James Crandell, statistician at the University of North Carolina at Chapel Hill, proposed a method for synthesising qualitative and quantitative research using Bayesian statistics. In Bayes' theorem, named after eighteenth-century statistician Thomas Bayes, the probability of a hypothesis is modified by emerging evidence, thus shifting from prior to posterior probability. For fusion of qualitative and quantitative evidence, Crandell and colleagues [10] advised that the findings from each paradigm should be analysed together. Testing their model in a review of adherence to HIV medication, they categorised similar themes and outcomes into ten variables (e.g. side effects) and represented the findings with a numerical scale from 0 to 1. For the 15 quantitative studies, Cohen's d, a standardised difference between means, was used [11]. The effect size was rated as 0 if related to non-adherence, and as 1 if related to adherence, with a midpoint of 0.5 for uncertain or no relationship. The same scale was used for the 12 qualitative studies, and all ratings were placed in a matrix.

The Bayesian method by Crandell and associates is too advanced to describe here, but for illustrative purpose, the combined analysis of qualitative and quantitative findings produced the following results for the ten variables (Table 9.1):

This type of analysis is philosophically contentious, and the mixed-method reviewer should proceed with caution. There is a subtle (some may say obvious) positivist orientation in combining the two sets of findings. Qualitative studies do not normally deal with 'variables, 'outcomes and 'results. However, this is an interesting development in mixed-method synthesis. For further reading on transforming study findings to an effect size amenable to statistical analysis, we suggest Sawilowsky [12] and Ferguson [13].

Table 9.1 Point estimates and posterior credible intervals from Bayesian data augmentation algorithm

Factor		Posterior mean (with 95% credible interval)
Relating to adherence	Belief that antiretroviral medication might do good	0.96 (0.90–1.0)
	Positive social network	0.85 (0.76–0.94)
	Routinisation	0.80 (0.60–0.98)
Relating to neither	Having or living with children	0.64 (0.45–0.83)
	Healthy or low virologic load	0.62 (0.29–0.90)
Relating to non-adherence	More complex regimen	0.29 (0.11–0.48)
	Disclosure/stigma/threats to confidentiality	0.21 (0.07–0.36)
	Side effects	0.21 (0.09–0.32)
	Negative feelings	0.19 (0.10–0.29)
	Belief that antiretroviral medication might do harm	0.16 (0.08–0.25)

Noting a tendency for mixed-method reviewers to favour a positivist or interpretivist approach, Sandelowski and colleagues at the University of North Carolina at Chapel Hill [14] urged a shift in focus from methods to the findings of studies. Applying the logic of synthesis, it is not the form but the content that is most important:

> Reviewers must, for example, be willing to see the reasons a group of people gave for missing medication doses produced from a thematic analysis of data generated from open-ended and minimally structured interviews with a purposefully selected sample of participants as potentially comparable to the predictors of missed doses produced from a regression analysis of data generated from closed-ended and highly structured questionnaires completed by a probability sample of participants.

9.5 Divergent Findings

A common occurrence with a mixed-method study or review is divergence between qualitative and quantitative data or findings. It is the responsibility of the researcher or reviewer to explore and offer an explanation for such differences. The process of aggregation combines thematically similar findings, while configuration deals with thematically dissimilar findings. As a political analogy, aggregation is a democratic verdict, while configuration takes account of minority groups. There is strength in number, but a mixed-method reviewer should beware a tyranny of the majority.

In the evaluation model of Pawson and Tilley [15], a mixed-method design can show how and why groups of people differ in their response to an intervention. An example in their book *Realistic Evaluation* demonstrated an opposite effect between groups. A local smoking cessation campaign featured posters in workplaces and other communal areas, such that it was impossible for people to miss the message. Results of the campaign showed that it reduced smoking among light and moderate smokers; heavy smokers, by contrast, indulged in their habit as frequently as ever (some smoked more).

One of this book's authors saw a stark contrast between qualitative and quantitative data in an evaluation of a service redevelopment [16]. In a 2-year programme, the hitherto disparate mental health services for older people in a London borough were integrated. A major component of the evaluation was staff morale: did the programme help or hinder their practice?, and did it improve relationships? NM conducted qualitative interviews with each member of staff and distributed a standardised instrument to measure work satisfaction. The data went in opposite directions: questionnaire results showed improved satisfaction, while interview findings conveyed discontent.

Based on close contact with the teams over a lengthy period, McCrea and Banerjee believed that the truth was somewhere between these two positions. The work satisfaction scale was completed three times during the programme, and results were presented at feedback meetings for all staff. After the first presentation, the team with lowest satisfaction scores drew attention. Team members felt that they were being portrayed negatively by other staff, and the team manager was understandably concerned. This team's ratings jumped up to above average in the next set of results. A similar change occurred with the team that was rated lowest in the second presentation. Overall, results improved in every team over the series.

Two phases of interviews were conducted, at the start and end of the programme. In the first interviews, participants displayed enthusiasm for their work and appreciated the interest shown by management. They seemed to enjoy talking about their work to an interested listener, over a 1-hour appointment. Much of the interview was used to explain what they do, with anecdotes of interesting and rewarding experiences. In the second interviews, participants focused on undesirable aspects of their work and relationships, often of limited relevance to the programme. In retrospect, McCrae and Banerjee believed that members of staff were using the interviews to pass messages to management. Only talking about the positives would have been a wasted opportunity.

McCrae and Banerjee suspected social desirability bias in the quantitative data and exploit of the interviews to seek better conditions. Any complex intervention in healthcare is likely to be influenced by the attitudes, perceptions and motives of the people involved and a plethora of contextual factors unrelated to the intervention. In their evaluation model, Pawson and Tilley explained that the investigator's task is to determine *what works*, *for whom* and *in what circumstances*, as depicted by this formula

$$\text{Context} \rightarrow \text{Mechanism} \rightarrow \text{Outcome}$$

However, a problem of any systematic review is that the findings are necessarily removed from the context of the study. This can be mitigated by presenting 'text in context', whereby findings are accompanied by contextual information that are necessary to fully understand the phenomenon [14]. This could include details of the participants, their setting and the time of data collection in relation to a studied intervention or experience.

9.6   Conclusion

A mixed-method review is not for the faint-hearted, and it may be advisable for a novice to limit a review to one paradigm. In our experience many students naively attempt 'thematic analysis' of studies with a mixture of statistical and interpretative findings, but this should not be done unless the reviewer has a clear understanding of the meaning of 'theme' and a rationale for converting quantitative results to a qualitative formulation. As well as considerable practical challenges, combining qualitative and quantitative findings is problematic due to conflicting ontological stances.

Nonetheless, there are some study topics for which a more inclusive approach is justified. Evaluation of a complex intervention, such as a new model of service, is likely to be concerned with both process and outcomes. A mix of qualitative and quantitative information may be needed to understand *how* an intervention is experienced, as well as its performance on predetermined outcome measures. Instead of seeking precision, the mixed-method reviewer sees diversity as strength. Perhaps the best term to represent such endeavour is not a matrix but a mosaic.

References

1. Midgley M (1989) Wisdom, information, and wonder: what is knowledge for? Routledge, London, New York
2. Greenhalgh T (2018) How to implement evidence-based healthcare. Wiley, Hoboken, NJ
3. Wootton D (2016) Invention of science. HarperCollins Publishers, New York
4. Guba EG, Lincoln YS (1991) Effective evaluation: improving the usefulness of evaluation results through responsive and naturalistic approaches. Jossey-Bass Publishers, San Francisco
5. Hammersley M (1996) The relationship between qualitative and quantitative research: paradigm loyalty versus methodological eclecticism. In: Richardson JTE, Richardson JTE (eds) Handbook of qualitative research methods for psychology and the social sciences. British Psychological Society, Leicester, pp 159–174
6. Tashakkori A, Teddlie C (1998) Mixed methodology: combining qualitative and quantitative approaches. Sage, Thousand Oaks, CA
7. Sandelowski M, Voils CI, Barroso J (2006) Defining and designing mixed research synthesis studies. Res Sch 13:29
8. Jordan Z, Lockwood C, Munn Z, Aromataris E (2019) The updated Joanna Briggs Institute model of evidence-based healthcare. Int J Evid Based Healthc 17:58–71. https://doi.org/10.1097/XEB.0000000000000155
9. Lizarondo L, Stern C, Carrier J, Godfrey C, Rieger K, Salmond S, Apostolo J, Kirkpatrick P, Loveday H (2020) Chapter 8: Mixed methods systematic reviews. In: Aromataris E, Munn Z (eds) JBI Manual for evidence synthesis. JBI. Available from https://wiki.jbi.global/display/MANUAL/Chapter+8%3A+Mixed+methods+systematic+reviews. https://doi.org/10.46658/JBIMES-20-09
10. Crandell JL, Voils CI, Chang Y, Sandelowski M (2011) Bayesian data augmentation methods for the synthesis of qualitative and quantitative research findings. Qual Quant 45:653–669. https://doi.org/10.1007/s11135-010-9375-z
11. Cohen J (1988) Statistical power analysis for the behavioral sciences, 2nd edn. L. Erlbaum Associates, Hillsdale, NJ
12. Sawilowsky SS (2009) New effect size rules of thumb. J Mod Appl Stat Meth 8:597–599. https://doi.org/10.22237/jmasm/1257035100
13. Ferguson CJ (2009) An effect size primer: a guide for clinicians and researchers. Prof Psychol Res Pract 40:532–538. https://doi.org/10.1037/a0015808
14. Sandelowski M, Voils CI, Leeman J, Crandell JL (2012) Mapping the mixed methods–mixed research synthesis terrain. J Mixed Methods Res 6:317–331. https://doi.org/10.1177/1558689811427913
15. Pawson R, Tilley N (1997) Realistic evaluation. Sage, London, Thousand Oaks, CA
16. McCrae N, Banerjee S (2011) Modernizing mental health services for older people: a case study. Int Psychogeriatr 23:10–19. https://doi.org/10.1017/S1041610210001407

Meaning and Implications: The Discussion

10

Summary Learning Points

- The discussion should contain a statement of principal findings but not repeat all of them, consider what does the reader need to know?
- The strengths and weaknesses of the review should be considered, including both the literature and the review process.
- The meaning of the review findings should be explained, remember the key audience is normally the nonexpert but interested reader who wants to learn about the subject, so make this accessible.
- The implications for practice, policy and research should be made clear.
- Any recommendation should clearly come from the data, and the logic of how these translate should be clear.
- The quality of the body of evidence, as well as the risk of bias of the review should be considered.
- The review should be presented using the appropriate reporting guidance.

By the time that you start the discussion, you are well on the way to completing your systematic review. But you cannot relax yet. The discussion is the vital section in which you present the meaning and implications of your review. Perhaps more than in any other part of your report, the discussion relies on writing skill. There is art and science in making sense of your findings, as you integrate the internal material (your results) with the external (the wider context of evidence, policy and practice). Ideally, you will be able to show how your review has enhanced understanding of the topic.

The word 'discussion' may be confusing. Its traditional dictionary definition is to 'debate; examine by argument' [1, p. 158]. Importantly, 'argument' in the context of a literature review does not mean having a row, or stubbornly defending a personal position or opinion, but rather 'examining agreements and disagreements with other studies or reviews' on the same or similar questions [2]. Discussing your review is quite different to an academic essay or personal blog. It is not about your personal beliefs but a rational, evidence-based defence of your review (the evidence, of course, is your findings).

© The Editor(s) (if applicable) and The Author(s), under exclusive license to Springer Nature Switzerland AG 2020
E. Purssell, N. McCrae, *How to Perform a Systematic Literature Review*,
https://doi.org/10.1007/978-3-030-49672-2_10

Watson [3], editor of the *Journal of Advanced Nursing*, remarked:

In my work around the world, delivering 'writing for publication' workshops, a frequent question is: 'How do you start writing the discussion section of a manuscript?' The question is not 'How do you write the discussion?' but: 'How do you start?'

The answer to this is that the discussion should start by summarising the main results of the review, in no more than an opening paragraph. Erroneously, some writers use the discussion to repeat the results in detail, or reveal new information from the data, which should have been described in the previous section of the report. This is not the place for internal comparisons but for showing what your review adds to the evidence base and its implications for practice, policy and further research.

Guidance here is provided by the Centre for Reviews and Dissemination (CRD), whose *Guidance for Undertaking Reviews in Healthcare* [4] recommends that a discussion should contain the following:

• Statement of principal findings
• Strengths and weaknesses of the review
• Meaning of the review findings
• Implications

10.1   Statement of Findings

Before presenting the main outcomes of the review, you should remind readers of the purpose of the work. For example, 'this systematic review analysed and synthesised evidence from empirical studies of the influence of social media on adolescent mental health'. Immediately following this introductory sentence, you should present the key findings. Instead of restating the entire set of results, summarise the outcomes that answer the review question.

We have emphasised throughout that statistical significance is not the same as clinical significance, and this is a good place to re-emphasise that point. While statistical significance can be judged from the p-value and confidence interval, clinical significance is more nuanced; it is a judgement that should be based on rational argument. The ability to make this kind of argument is what marks you out as an expert in the area. Neither of us as authors have expertise in dermatology, but we could read a study report on treatment of psoriasis and assess the statistical significance of the findings with ease. We would be not so sure of the clinical significance.

You may have enough knowledge to assess clinical significance or you could consult experts in the field. You may also ask patients what would be significant to them: a new drug that prolongs life by a year may be worth taking despite side effects, but perhaps not if the difference is only a week. Patient and public involvement, as recommended in the design and conduct of primary research, is becoming increasingly important in systematic reviews too and is vital if you are to make clinical recommendations. You should not really make clinical recommendations without the involvement of patients or service users.

You should relate your findings to the context of existing literature. How does your review differ, and what is its contribution to knowledge? There is nothing inherently wrong with subjectivity; you have completed a comprehensive review of the relevant literature, and so you have earned the right to interpret the findings. However, you should differentiate fact from opinion (unlike some politicians!). Take care not to indulge in 'spin and boasting' [5], which is to overstate your findings while denigrating those who have come before. Admitting to 'committing some of these literary sins' in the past, Cummings and Rivara emphasised that while there are pitfalls to avoid, 'improving writing is a lifelong process'. This is a conclusion with which we would concur, and note that this book has been through many drafts before publication; sometimes students expect their work to be perfect straight away.

10.1.1 Efficacy or Effectiveness

When relating your findings to practice, it is important to be clear about the difference between efficacy and effectiveness. Efficacy can be defined as the extent to which an intervention does more good than harm in ideal conditions, as in controlled trials; think of it as answering the question: 'can it work?' Effectiveness, by contrast, is a question of whether an intervention does more good than harm in real conditions: 'does it work in practice?' [6, p. 652]. Often we find that people erroneously believe that they are looking at effectiveness when they have RCTs that are very different in context to normal practice.

Here we see a major limitation in rigid hierarchies of research methods. While RCTs are rightly considered to be a high level of evidence, they usually test efficacy rather than effectiveness. Imagine you are testing a new drug for heart failure, named EdMed. Your trial is likely to exclude the sickest patients and those with comorbidities; they will be given the best available current treatment, as it would be unethical to treat them with an experimental drug of unknown effect. The trial is likely to be very structured with strict dosing regimens. EdMed may appear to be a great success, but the patients who probably need treatment the most, those who are sickest, were not included in your trial, and EdMed might have a different effect in this group. When EdMed is approved, these may well be the very first to be offered this new and expensive drug. Thus the context of the RCT is very different from the context of practice. Here we see one of the many dilemmas in creating and using evidence: the highly controlled world of the RCT is great for minimising bias and controlling the influence of confounding variables; but it is these very features that preclude assessment of its real-world impact in the form of effectiveness.

There is one caveat to this. If the context of the study is very similar to real life, a RCT could show effectiveness. Sometimes you may hear people refer to 'pragmatic' trials [7], which may have less stringent eligibility criteria, more flexibility in the intervention and other features that make them less like and RCT and more like clinical practice, or practice itself may be very controlled, just like the study. Observational studies on the other hand, which are lower in the hierarchy of evidence have less control, but are able to show real-world impact and so are more likely to show effectiveness. The irony is that the high level of control that makes RCTs a high level of evidence is the very reason that means they usually don't show effectiveness—which is what people usually want to know!

Alongside efficacy and effectiveness, there is a third 'e': efficiency, which considers the effect of an intervention in relation to the resources it consumes [6, p. 652]. For efficiency of the intervention, the question will be: 'is it worth doing?' We will not be considering the complexities of cost-benefit analysis in detail here, but the costs of a treatment include both clinical costs and financial cost, and we will be returning to this later when we discuss decision-making in the context of GRADE.

If you struggled with the idea of a discussion, hopefully this section alone will help you to see its importance. The task is much more complicated than summarising research findings, placing the studies in a hierarchy of evidence and coming to a conclusion. If that is all it took anyone with a basic research understanding could do it. Clinical context is everything!

10.2   Strengths and Weaknesses of the Review

No review is perfect. By noting limitations, you are not undermining your work, but taking the opportunity to demonstrate scientific proficiency. What could have been done differently to improve the review (perhaps if you had more time or resources)? Your report, whether submitted as an academic assignment or to a journal, will be examined by people who will look for errors of commission and omission. So get your excuses in first!

There are two main tools that you can use (and others may also use) to judge the quality of your review, these are AMSTAR 2, a critical appraisal tool; and ROBIS, a risk of bias tool. There is also a CASP tool for systematic reviews which will not be discussed further here, but it follows the same principles as the other CASP tools mentioned in previous chapters. Just to put this into context, you may remember in Chap. 5 that we said that there really is no single meaning of quality in research but rather four related but distinct types. Here we are interested in assessment of the first three types of quality assessment at review level only; plus the fourth, which is review-specific:

- Quality of reporting of the individual studies and of the review
- Quality of the conduct or methodology of the individual studies and of the review
- Risk of bias of the individual studies and of the review
- Quality of the total body of evidence in the review

10.2.1   Critical Appraisal: AMSTAR 2

AMSTAR 2 (A Measurement Tool to Assess Systematic Reviews) is a critical appraisal tool for systematic reviews of randomised and nonrandomised studies [8]. Following on from the original AMSTAR (hence the 2), the new version has 16 items of which 7 are thought to be critical. The possible answers are yes or no, where yes indicates a positive response; if there is insufficient information, this should lead to a no answer apart from a few questions where partial yes is a possibility. Assessing each question in this way allows you to come to the conclusion about the overall confidence in the results of the review. These are high if there are no weaknesses or one noncritical weakness; moderate if there is more than one non-critical weakness; low if there is one critical flaw with or without noncritical weaknesses; or critically low if there is more than one critical flaw with or without noncritical weaknesses. The implication of this last rating is that the review is critically flawed and is not likely to be an accurate and comprehensive summary of the research literature.

10.2.2   Risk of Bias: ROBIS

ROBIS (Risk of Bias Assessment Tool for Systematic Reviews) is a tool for assessing the risk of bias in systematic reviews [9] and so is the review level equivalent of the Cochrane RoB2 or ROBINS-I. It consists of three phases, the first of which is an optional first phase to assess relevance, that is, did the review answer the question that the authors asked in the first place? The second phase is much like RoB2 and ROBINS-I, this time with four domains and a number of signalling questions for each of these domains. Each of the signalling questions can be answered in one of five ways: yes or no, probably yes or no, or no information, where yes indicates a low risk of bias. Therefore the greater the number of answers that are answered negatively, the greater the risk of bias. The third and final phase consists of a judgement about the risk of bias in the systematic review as a whole. The structure of this is similar to the previous phase, using signalling questions to ascertain whether the concerns identified in the last phase have been addressed by the authors in their interpretation of the findings. If there are no concerns, or if concerns have been appropriately considered, the overall assessment may be that there is a low risk of bias. This phase also considers matters relating to the interpretation of the review findings.

The decision for the review consists of coming to a conclusion about each of the two phases, possible judgements for each being: high concern, low concern or unclear concern, although the interpretation differs for each phase. For the first optional phase, high concern reflects a judgement that studies which are important and relevant to the review question are likely to have been excluded from the review, while for the second phase, it indicates that the synthesis is likely to have produced biased results. ROBIS and AMSTAR 2 are compared in Table 10.1.

Table 10.1 ROBIS and AMSTAR 2 compared

ROBIS domains	AMSTAR 2 critical domains
	Protocol registered before commencement of the review (item 2)
	Adequacy of the literature search (item 4)
Study eligibility criteria	Justification for excluding individual studies (item 7)
Identification and selection of studies	
Data collection and study appraisal	
	Risk of bias from individual studies being included in the review (item 9)
Synthesis and findings	Appropriateness of meta-analytical methods (item 11)
	Consideration of risk of bias when interpreting the results of the review (item 13)
	Assessment of presence and likely impact of publication bias (item 15)

10.3 Making Recommendations

As healthcare is a practical domain, it is likely that you will use your review findings to make clinical recommendations. However, making recommendations is contentious, because a review rarely involves the most important group of people—patients. The views of patients (and families if appropriate) are of the utmost importance in making clinical recommendations.

Apart from keeping patients at the centre of our consideration, the other key to making sound recommendations is that the process of deciding upon and wording them should be transparent, that is, to say it should be clear to readers how you went from the evidence in your review to the recommendations that you make at the end. To do this, we are going to use a system devised by the Grading of Recommendations, Assessment, Development and Evaluation Working Group, more commonly known as GRADE [10]. They have created a logical process for this task. The steps of the GRADE process that are relevant for us here are firstly assessing the quality of the evidence for the outcome of interest and then using four key criteria to decide the direction and the strength of a recommendation regarding it.

10.4 Assessing the Quality of Quantitative Evidence: GRADE

For quantitative reviews, the evidence regarding an outcome will usually comprise either randomised controlled trial evidence or nonrandomised study evidence which would include observational studies. If you look at the hierarchy of evidence, you will see that RCTs are at the top, and other types of study lower down. However, unlike the traditional hierarchy, GRADE is more flexible. It allows for lower-quality RCT evidence to be downgraded and higher-quality observational evidence to be upgraded, meaning that high-quality observational or nonrandomised evidence might actually be better than lower-quality RCT evidence. Quality in this context is defined as 'the extent to which our confidence in an estimate of the effect is adequate to support a particular recommendation' [10].

There are five reasons why you might reduce the evidence provided by randomised controlled trials:

1. *Risk of bias*—bias is a systematic error, or deviation from the truth, essentially answering the question do you think based on the method used that the results are likely to be right? This is considered both at the study level and the outcome level using tools such as the Cochrane ROB2 and ROBINS-I and is discussed in detail in Chap. 6.
2. *Inconsistency*—this refers to differences or heterogeneity in the underlying effects of the studies. You may recall there are three types of heterogeneity: clinical, methodological and outcome. Although researchers tend to concentrate on the last of these, they are all important and should be considered. This is discussed in detail in Chap. 7.
3. *Indirectness*—generally the best evidence consists of direct comparisons between treatments and conducted with a population and in a context similar to that in which the recommendation will be implemented. If this is not the case you have indirectness of the evidence.
4. *Imprecision*—remembering that quantitative research normally aims to take results from a sample and to apply them to a population, here we are concerned with the precision of that estimate of the population parameter. This is normally assessed using the confidence interval, with a wide interval showing imprecision.
5. *Publication bias*—there is evidence that some types of study are more likely than other to be published. If, for example those with positive results are more likely to be published than those with negative results, the estimate of overall effect may be inaccurate or wrong.

Each of these will reduce the strength of evidence provided by a body of evidence.

There are also three reasons for upgrading the evidence from nonrandomised or observational studies:

1. *Large magnitude of an effect*—if the result was very high, the response very good, or the relationship very strong; this might increase your confidence that it is real.
2. *Dose-response gradient*—sometimes you will see a relationship between the amount of something and the resultant effect. For example, if there is a relationship between the drug dosages and outcomes, this might again increase your confidence that this effect is real.
3. *Effect of plausible residual confounding*—if there are there other confounding factors that mean the thing you are interested in should not work, but it still does, then again this might increase your confidence in this result.

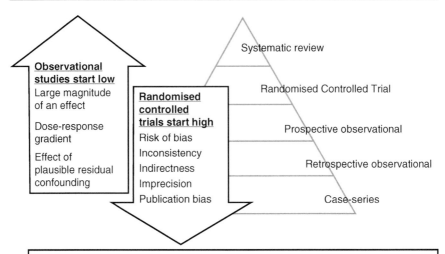

High confidence - Further research is very unlikely to change our confidence in the estimate of effect.

Moderate confidence - Further research is likely to have an important impact on our confidence in the estimate of effect and may change the estimate.

Low confidence - Further research is very likely to have an important impact on our confidence in the estimate of effect and is likely to change estimate.

Very low confidence - Any estimate of effect is very uncertain.

For each factor that leads to downgrading, this can be by one or two levels. Large magnitude of effect can lead to upgrading by one or two levels, the other two factors can lead to upgrading by one level.

Fig. 10.1 Assessing quantitative evidence using GRADE

Each of these will increase the strength of evidence provided by a body of evidence.

These are shown in Fig. 10.1.

10.5   Assessing the Quality of Qualitative Evidence: GRADE CERQual

The criteria for assessing a body of evidence above relate to quantitative research. For qualitative research there is an equivalent called GRADE-CERQual, which is short for Confidence in the Evidence from Reviews of Qualitative Research [11]. A more recent innovation that the original GRADE tools, it is not perhaps as well developed as GRADE and certainly has a smaller body of supporting literature. CERQual is based on the idea of assessing confidence in the review findings, defined as 'an assessment of the extent to which a review finding is a reasonable representation of the phenomenon of interest' [12, p. 1].

The assessment of the evidence supporting a finding starts off with review findings starting off by as high confidence which can then be rated down on the basis of four criteria; there is a fifth *dissemination bias*, but this is yet to be fully adopted [12].

1. *Methodological limitations*—this refers to whether there are concerns about the design or conduct of the individual studies in the review that are used to support a finding.
2. *Coherence*—asks how clear, well supported and compelling is the fit is between the data from the individual studies and a review finding that comes from them.
3. *Adequacy of data*—the quantity and degree of richness that supports a finding.
4. *Relevance*—this assesses how applicable the context of the studies is to that in the review question, for example, how similar are the perspectives, populations, phenomena of interest and setting.
5. *Dissemination bias*—this refers to the systematic distortion of the phenomenon of interest in a finding as a result of selectivity in the dissemination of studies. It is similar to publication bias. This does not currently form part of CERQual; it is under development [13].

These criteria give an assessment of the confidence that we can have in the quality of the evidence, remembering that for GRADE this means the extent to which an 'estimate of the effect is adequate to support a particular recommendation' for guidelines, and the 'extent to which we are confident that an estimate of the effect is correct' for systematic reviews [10]. For CERQual, it means 'an assessment of the extent to which a review finding is a reasonable representation of the phenomenon of interest' [12, p. 14]. This is shown in Fig. 10.2.

10.6 Turning Evidence into Recommendations

Assessment of confidence in the review evidence is one of the four GRADE criteria that are used to develop findings in a transparent way. These are shown in Table 10.2. You will note that this includes the patient's values and preferences, which you will only know if you have patient representatives or other evidence in the review team. While this is the case for well-formulated guideline development groups, it is not the case for most systematic review teams; hence strictly speaking, systematic reviews should only make clinical recommendations with caveats.

A sometimes crucial consideration in making recommendations is resource implications. The writer Thomas Carlyle said in the nineteenth century that economics is 'the dismal science', if this is the case, then health economics is probably the dismalist end of this because health interventions and their effects are so hard to cost and quantify. For example, you can cost a thermometer fairly easily, and that it takes 3 min to take a temperature, but hospitals probably negotiate their own prices, and then you need to add in staff costs for the time to take a temperature while taking into account other things that nurses might do while also taking a

Fig. 10.2
Assessing qualitative
evidence using
GRADE CERqual

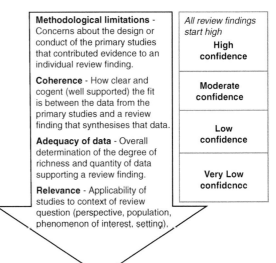

Methodological limitations - Concerns about the design or conduct of the primary studies that contributed evidence to an individual review finding.

Coherence - How clear and cogent (well supported) the fit is between the data from the primary studies and a review finding that synthesises that data.

Adequacy of data - Overall determination of the degree of richness and quantity of data supporting a review finding.

Relevance - Applicability of studies to context of review question (perspective, population, phenomenon of interest, setting).

All review findings start high
High confidence

Moderate confidence

Low confidence

Very Low confidcncc

High confidence - It is highly likely that the review finding is a reasonable representation of the phenomenon of interest
Moderate confidence - It is likely that the review finding is a reasonable representation of the phenomenon of interest
Low confidence - It is possible that the review finding is a reasonable representation of the phenomenon of interest
Very low confidence - It is not clear whether the review finding is a reasonable representation of the phenomenon of interest.

There is a fifth criterion - **dissemination bias** which is defined as systematic distortion of the phenomenon of interest due to selective dissemination of studies or individual study findings. This has yet to be fully implemented within CERQual

Table 10.2   GRADE criteria for giving strength to a recommendation

GRADE criterion	Explanation
What confidence can we have in the estimate of patient's values and preferences (the quality of the evidence)	If the evidence is strong, it is more likely that a strong recommendation will be made. For this use, the GRADE or GRADE CERQual criteria
What is the balance between the desirable and undesirable outcomes of the recommendation?	Most recommended actions will have positive and negative effects which need to be balanced. Drugs, for example, will have the intended positive effects but will also have negative side effects. Think about the overall balance, does it have a net positive or negative balance?
What confidence do we have in the patient's values and preferences?	If there is a lot of variation or uncertainty about what patients want, this might reduce the strength of any recommendation. This should be based on patient and wider stakeholder involvement
What are the resource implications?	If a recommended action is very expensive, it is less likely that a strong recommendation will be made

temperature. For example, the nurse might take a blood pressure and pulse, talk to the patient and maybe even have a tidy-up of the area they are in. Should these be added in? If you do want to try this, a good place to start if you are in the UK is the Unit Costs of Health and Social Care (https://www.pssru.ac.uk/project-pages/unit-costs/). If you are not in the UK, it might be worth finding out if your country has a similar publication. You may be surprised by how much many things (including maybe yourself!) cost.

Patient and public involvement is key to guideline development, but not normally systematic reviews, which is why GRADE does not include the latter in the recommendation process. The National Institute for Health and Care Excellence (NICE), for example, require that lay people or patients and organisations representing them are involved in the guideline development process [14]. You may also find evidence about patient preferences, although in most areas of healthcare, this is either absent or not very strong. Incidentally great care needs to be taken to ensure that this is not just a tokenistic process; lay representatives may require training and assistance, and it needs to be made clear that they are the equal of everyone else in the team.

In addition to these 'core' criteria, the World Health Organization [15] suggests that you might need to consider four more criteria:

1. The importance or priority of the problem being addressed
2. Equity and human rights
3. Acceptability
4. Feasibility

The possible outcomes from this are five different types of recommendation and the possibility of good practice points. The recommendations have two features, a direction for or against something and a strength. The strength is based on what proportion of people who form the population to which the recommendation is to be applied would want the proposed course of action. Note that even in the case of a strong recommendation, it does not mean that everyone would want it.

A more detailed version of the GRADE criteria for giving strength to recommendations are given in the evidence-to-decision frameworks, which have been developed for different types of question, and in some cases for individual and population-level decisions. Table 10.3 shows the criteria for these when considering questions of effectiveness [16, 17].

Sometimes there is no evidence for a healthcare activity, but you have practical experience. As you know, expert opinion is not really a form of evidence (it is an expert *interpretation* of evidence), but nonetheless we sometimes use it to make recommendations. We call these good practice points (GPP); these are recommendations for best practice based on the experience of the guideline development group. They characteristically represent situations in which a large and compelling body of indirect evidence, made up of linked evidence including several indirect comparisons, strongly supports the net benefit of the recommended action [18]. These are shown in Table 10.4.

Table 10.3 GRADE evidence-to-decision framework

Population perspective	Individual patient perspective
Is the problem a priority (from a population perspective)?	Is the problem a priority (from the perspective of individual patients)?
How substantial are the desirable anticipated effects?	
How substantial are the undesirable anticipated effects?	
What is the overall certainty of the evidence of effects?	
Is there important uncertainty about or variability in how much people value the main outcomes?	
Does the balance between desirable and undesirable effects favour the intervention or the comparison?	
How large are the resource requirements (costs)?	Does the cost-effectiveness of the intervention (the out-of-pocket cost relative to the net desirable effect) favour the intervention or the comparison?
What is the certainty of the evidence of resource requirements (costs)?	
Does the cost-effectiveness of the intervention favour the intervention or the comparison?	
What would be the impact on health equity?	
Is the intervention acceptable to key stakeholders?	Is the intervention acceptable to patients, their care givers and healthcare providers?
Is the intervention feasible to implement?	Is the intervention feasible for patients, their care givers and healthcare providers?

Table 10.4 Strengths of recommendations and their wording

Strong recommendation for	Weak recommendation for	No recommendation	Weak recommendation against	Strong recommendation against
A strong recommendation implies that most individuals in this situation would want the recommended course of action, and only a small number would not.				
These use words or phrases such as *we recommend that...* or *clinicians should/should not...* or words such as *do...*, *don't...*				
A weak recommendation implies that the majority of individuals in this situation would want the suggested course of action but also that many would not.				
These recommendations should use less certain wording, for example, *we suggest...* or *clinicians might.*				
Good practice points are recommendations based on experience or a large body of indirect evidence				

Returning to the meta-analysis that we performed in Chap. 7, we can now decide using these criteria whether or not to recommend antibiotics for a sore throat. The quality of evidence is quite strong, with a low risk of bias accross the studies. The values and preferences that patients have would be variable, do you think that they are likely to want antibiotics and how strong is the evidence for this? The variability probably means quite weak. The resource implications may be signficant because although often not expensive, if a large number of people desire antibiotics overall this may be very costly. However when you add in the balance of desirable and undesirable effects the decision becomes clearer; the effect is probably not clinically significant and there are many undesirable effects of treating sore throats with antibiotics, most notably antiboitic resistance.

We can now proceed to thinking about recommendations from patients' perspective. Based on the results of the meta-analysis alone, we can see there is evidence for antibiotics being effective in reducing the number of people with a sore throat, but when these other issues are considered, we can understand the reason for making a strong recommendation *against* taking antibiotics for a sore throat. Most individuals, given this information, would want the recommended course of action (i.e. to not have antibiotics), and only a small number would not. This is despite the quite high-quality evidence in our meta-analysis that they are effective in reducing sore throats. This reflects the UK guidance, which states that for those with are unlikely to benefit from antibiotics as they have a low risk of having streptococcal infection (defined as less than 17–18% depending upon the tool used), the recommendation is 'Do not offer an antibiotic prescription' [19]. If you look at the wording in Table 10.4, you will see the wording of a strong recommendation, compared to that for people with a higher risk, where the recommendation is 'Consider no antibiotic prescription with advice'.

10.7   Evidence Profiles and Summary of Findings Table

Two of the key features of the GRADE process are the evidence profile and summary of findings table. The evidence profile is a detailed quality assessment including an explicit judgment for each factor within GRADE that determines the quality of evidence for each outcome, while the summary is similar but without the detailed judgements. The reason for having these two different tables is that they are really aimed at different audiences, with most readers only really being concerned with the summary [20]. Summary of findings tables have seven elements, not all of which will be applicable in all cases, but you should consider them [21, 22].

1. A list of all important outcomes, both those which are desirable and those which are undesirable.
2. A measure of the 'typical burden' of these outcomes, for example, the result in the control group, or estimated risk. This shows the baseline level before the intervention is put in place.
3. A measure of the risk in the intervention group or a measure of the difference between the risks with and without intervention. In the case of continuous outcomes, this could be the mean difference or standardised mean difference showing the change associated with intervention.
4. The relative magnitude of effect, which could include the relative risk or odds ratio.
5. The numbers of studies and participants contributing to the assessment of the outcome.
6. A rating of the overall confidence in effect estimates for each outcome (which may vary by outcome).
7. Any comments.

Both types of table can be produced using GRADEPro as outlined in Appendix B.

10.8 Establishing Confidence in the Output of Qualitative Research Synthesis

For appraising the findings of a review of qualitative research, you may use ConQual, which is a member of the Joanna Briggs Institute (JBI) family of methods [23], as mentioned in Chap. 5. If you have been using the JBI tools throughout, you should use ConQual. This looks very similar to CERQual; the authors suggest that the main point of difference is that ConQual focuses on the credibility (internal validity) of the findings, whereas CERQual focuses on the plausibility or coherence (the fit between the data from the primary studies and the review finding) [12, 23]. CONQual could theoretically just be used with the above process using ConQual as a method of assessing the quality of the evidence in place of CERQual if desired (Fig. 10.3).

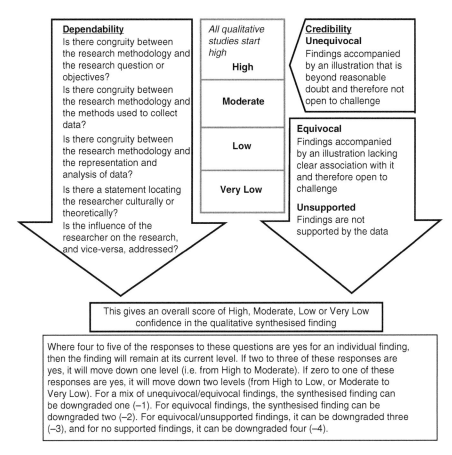

Fig. 10.3 Assessing qualitative evidence using JBI ConQual

10.9   Limitations of the Author

Healthcare practitioners are encouraged to reflect on their actions and attitudes, and this ability is useful for research too. You are not expected to self-flagellate, and we advise against statements such as 'the author is inexperienced in systematic reviewing' (or words to that effect). However, you should acknowledge the limitations of working on your own, as this could raise the risk of error and thus impair reliability. Remember reliability is a concept quite distinct from bias; reliability is random error, such as incorrectly copying down a number from a paper in the review or misinterpreting a finding. The need to reduce these errors is why we normally do this in duplicate. This is not merely of problem for the novice: Gøtzsche and colleagues [24] found numerous errors in published meta-analyses.

10.10   Conclusion

This chapter has shown how to make sense of the findings of a review and develop a discussion and then recommendations arising from the evidence. However, a review will be of limited value if it does not reach its intended audience. The final chapter, therefore, is concerned with making the most of your review and its implications.

References

1. Browning D (1942) Everyman's English Dictionary. JM Dent, London
2. Schünemann HJ, Visit GE, Higgins JP et al (2019) Chapter 15: Interpreting results and drawing conclusions. In: Higgins J, Thomas J, Chandler J et al (eds). Cochrane Handbook for Systematic Reviews of Interventions version 6.0 (updated July 2019), Cochrane, London. www.training.cochrane.org/handbook
3. Watson R (2018) Starting the "Discussion" section of a manuscript, nurse author and editor. http://naepub.com/reporting-research/2018-28-2-3/. Accessed 6 Mar 2020
4. Centre for Reviews and Dissemination (ed) (2009) CRD's guidance for undertaking reviews in healthcare, 3rd edn. York Publ. Services, York
5. Cummings P, Rivara FP (2012) Spin and boasting in research articles. Arch Pediatr Adolesc Med 166:1099. https://doi.org/10.1001/archpediatrics.2012.1461
6. Haynes B (1999) Can it work? Does it work? Is it worth it? BMJ 319:652–653. https://doi.org/10.1136/bmj.319.7211.652
7. Patsopoulos NA (2011) A pragmatic view on pragmatic trials. Dialogues Clin Neurosci 13:217–224
8. Shea BJ, Reeves BC, Wells G et al (2017) AMSTAR 2: a critical appraisal tool for systematic reviews that include randomised or non-randomised studies of healthcare interventions, or both. BMJ 358:j4008. https://doi.org/10.1136/bmj.j4008
9. Whiting P, Savović J, Higgins JPT et al (2016) ROBIS: a new tool to assess risk of bias in systematic reviews was developed. J Clin Epidemiol 69:225–234. https://doi.org/10.1016/j.jclinepi.2015.06.005

10. Schünemann H, Brożek J, Guyatt G, Oxman A (2013) GRADE handbook. https://gdt.gradepro.org/app/handbook/handbook.html. Accessed 6 Mar 2020

11. Lewin S, Glenton C, Munthe-Kaas H et al (2015) Using qualitative evidence in decision making for health and social interventions: an approach to assess confidence in findings from qualitative evidence syntheses (GRADE-CERQual). PLoS Med 12:e1001895. https://doi.org/10.1371/journal.pmed.1001895

12. Lewin S, Booth A, Glenton C et al (2018) Applying GRADE-CERQual to qualitative evidence synthesis findings: introduction to the series. Implement Sci 13:2. https://doi.org/10.1186/s13012-017-0688-3

13. Booth A, Lewin S, Glenton C et al (2018) Applying GRADE-CERQual to qualitative evidence synthesis findings—paper 7: understanding the potential impacts of dissemination bias. Implement Sci 13:12. https://doi.org/10.1186/s13012-017-0694-5

14. National Institute for Health and Care Excellence (2014) Patient and public involvement policy—Public Involvement Programme—Public involvement—NICE and the public—NICE Communities—About. In: NICE. https://www.nice.org.uk/about/nice-communities/nice-and-the-public/public-involvement/public-involvement-programme/patient-public-involvement-policy. Accessed 6 Mar 2020

15. World Health Organization (2014) WHO handbook for guideline development, 2nd edn. World Health Organization, Geneva. Available from https://apps.who.int/iris/handle/10665/145714

16. Alonso-Coello P, Oxman AD, Moberg J et al (2016a) GRADE Evidence to Decision (EtD) frameworks: a systematic and transparent approach to making well informed healthcare choices. 2: Clinical practice guidelines. BMJ 353:i2089. https://doi.org/10.1136/bmj.i2089

17. Alonso-Coello P, Schünemann HJ, Moberg J et al (2016b) GRADE Evidence to Decision (EtD) frameworks: a systematic and transparent approach to making well informed healthcare choices. 1: Introduction. BMJ 353:i2016. https://doi.org/10.1136/bmj.i2016

18. Guyatt GH, Schünemann HJ, Djulbegovic B, Akl EA (2015) Guideline panels should not GRADE good practice statements. J Clin Epidemiol 68:597–600. https://doi.org/10.1016/j.jclinepi.2014.12.011

19. National Institute of Health and Care Excellence (2018) Recommendations—Sore throat (acute): antimicrobial prescribing—Guidance—NICE. https://www.nice.org.uk/guidance/ng84/chapter/Recommendations#managing-acute-sore-throat. Accessed 6 Mar 2020

20. Guyatt G, Oxman AD, Akl EA et al (2011) GRADE guidelines: 1. Introduction—GRADE evidence profiles and summary of findings tables. J Clin Epidemiol 64:383–394. https://doi.org/10.1016/j.jclinepi.2010.04.026

21. Guyatt GH, Oxman AD, Santesso N et al (2013a) GRADE guidelines: 12. Preparing summary of findings tables—binary outcomes. J Clin Epidemiol 66:158–172. https://doi.org/10.1016/j.jclinepi.2012.01.012

22. Guyatt GH, Thorlund K, Oxman AD et al (2013b) GRADE guidelines: 13. Preparing summary of findings tables and evidence profiles—continuous outcomes. J Clin Epidemiol 66:173–183. https://doi.org/10.1016/j.jclinepi.2012.08.001

23. Munn Z, Porritt K, Lockwood C et al (2014) Establishing confidence in the output of qualitative research synthesis: the ConQual approach. BMC Med Res Methodol 14:108. https://doi.org/10.1186/1471-2288-14-108

24. Gøtzsche PC, Hróbjartsson A, Marić K, Tendal B (2007) Data extraction errors in meta-analyses that use standardized mean differences. JAMA 298:430–437. https://doi.org/10.1001/jama.298.4.430

Making an Impact: Dissemination of Results

11

Summary Learning Points

- For useful impact, findings of a systematic review need to be seen and applied in practice.
- A key decision is how to publish your review, in particular what journal? Take care when interpreting metrics such as impact factors as they can be very blunt tools and sometimes quite misleading.
- It is important to consider your target audience, where will they be likely to look.
- Open access publishing costs money but will increase the visibility of your review. Most non-open journals are not accessible to most people.
- You should put your paper in an institutional repository immediately upon acceptance but check the copyright restrictions.

We all want our work to be read and appreciated by others, and unlike the fate of many great artists who only gained recognition after their death, it would be nice if this came sooner rather than later. While rewards may range from a good mark in a course to transforming patient care depending on the purpose of the project and importance of the findings, everyone hopes to make a positive impact. The writer of a systematic review has an advantage because such a report is likely to be read more widely than that of a single study.

Research impact was first defined in the Research Excellence Framework [1] as the 'effect on, change or benefit to the economy, society, culture, public policy or services, health, the environment or quality of life, beyond academia'. The UK Research & Innovation Group [2] issued a similar definition:

> Impact is the demonstrable contribution that excellent research makes to society and the economy. This occurs in many ways—through creating and sharing new knowledge and innovation; inventing groundbreaking new products, companies and jobs; developing new and improving existing public services and policy; enhancing quality of life and health; and many more.

Impact on 'scientific advances, across and within disciplines' is differentiated from economic and societal impact, which includes 'benefit to individuals,

E. Purssell, N. McCrae, *How to Perform a Systematic Literature Review*, https://doi.org/10.1007/978-3-030-49672-2_11

organisations and nations' [2]. Most researchers would agree that the latter is more important than the former but also more difficult to measure. There is a persistent gap between theory and practice, and in a practical field such as healthcare, researchers should be aiming beyond a contribution to academic literature.

Time is important too. In the past, getting published in an academic journal was a slow process, but the Internet is a rocket that can send new research findings into cyberspace as soon as a paper is approved. Sadly, some journals have not kept pace with technological advances, incurring unnecessarily long periods between submission and publication. Evidence-based changes to practice will not happen while your review is with referees or 'in press', although many journals provide early view of accepted papers before a proof is published. Another challenge is the relentless growth in the number of journals, which has increased the competition for publicity. Will your review stand out from the crowd?

11.1   Making Your Review Relevant

When undertaking a systematic literature review, you may have included studies that do not readily apply to the context in which the results will be used. As discussed in Chap. 9, one of the criteria in the GRADE tool is indirectness, which occurs when there are differences between the interventions, populations or measures in the studies and your question. The TRANSFER approach was developed to enhance transferability, which is defined as 'an assessment of the degree to which the context of the review question and the context of studies contributing data to the review finding differ according to a priori identified characteristics (transfer factors)' [3, p. 2]. Put more simply, can the results be generalised to different settings? Assessment of this partly addresses one of the criticisms of reviews generally and meta-analysis more specifically that context is often removed from studies when presented in a review. Consider the forest plot presented in Chap. 6; this contains no significant contextual information at all, apart from the year of publication.

The TRANSFER process is quite complex. Ideally, it should be applied at the beginning of the review process, as it begins with a meeting with stakeholders prior to the review being undertaken to define the review question and context and then to decide on the characteristics (or transfer factors) that are likely to be important in assessing the fit between the question and the studies to be included in the review. Typically, around three to five tranfer factors may be determined. These decisions may inform the review process, for example, it might be that a particular country or geographical region has specific characteristics that make it necessary to do a separate analysis. You can then make an assessment as to the transferability of the review finding using the concerns for each of the individual transferability factors, the assessment being that there are no, minor, moderate or serious concerns. In Chap. 9, you will see that there are two GRADE criteria of particular relevance here: indirectness [4] and relevance [5].

Although you will probably not be able to go through this whole process unless you are on a large funded project, thinking about these transfer factors will allow you to apply your review to the specific context in which you are interested and also to consider contextual factors applicable in other settings. A comment that authors often get from peer reviewers on submitted papers is 'how does this apply in our/different countries or settings?' This is important because most journals have a global rather than national perspective.

11.2 Preparing for Publication

If the review is for an academic assignment, publication is a secondary objective. For doctoral study, one of the first tasks is the literature review, and this is often a good opportunity for publication. However, for students at any level, the format of an academic project will differ considerably from a submission to a journal. Do not underestimate the work needed to adapt the report of a review from one purpose to another.

When deciding where to seek publication of your paper, you should read each journal's instructions for authors carefully. Journals vary widely in what they will publish, how long papers can be, the structure of abstract, labelling of tables, hierarchy of headings and referencing style. If you don't follow these instructions carefully, your paper may be rejected by the editorial office before being seen by a member of the editorial team. Failing to follow the guidelines might suggest that you are careless or that your paper has already been submitted elsewhere. As well as following the rules, find some reviews already published in the journal and ensure that your writing is in tune with the house style. You may also need is a cover letter to the editor. These are not always required, but we would generally recommend this a courtesy. Typically a letter should state the title of the paper, explain briefly why it is important, confirm that all of the named authors have contributed to the paper and perhaps state what they did and assure that the paper has not been simultaneously submitted elsewhere. Submitting a paper to two peer-reviewed journals at the same time is unethical and likely to get you into trouble.

A potentially tricky decision is on authorship. Anyone named alongside you will share the credit for your work: do they deserve it? The Committee on Publication Ethics (commonly referred to as COPE) [6] states the minimum requirements for authorship as follows:

1. A substantial contribution to the work
2. Accountability for the work and its presentation in a publication

The conventional order of authors is for the first to be the writer, and the last as the chief investigator of the project or the academic supervisor. Simply being a manager or senior colleague does not fulfil point 1 above! Many journals also require information on what each author did towards the publication, to justify their listing.

The title and abstract are like a 'shop window'. These elements of your report have particular importance because they are searched by the bibliographic databases and are all that may be read by people who are considering whether the work is worth reading. Therefore, the title and abstract should be prepared with due care. A separate list of keywords is required by journals. One way of choosing keywords is to use the PubMed 'MeSH on demand' facility, which automatically finds MeSH terms relating to your text; otherwise, these may be identified and selected by using the MeSH browser directly. Just type in your keyword and see if there is a MeSH equivalent. Here you can look for the complete word using the 'FullWord Search' option (which is the default) or the 'SubString Search' which will also look for your term when embedded in another. For example, searching 'leukaemia' in the 'FullWord Search' retrieves leukaemia (as one would expect), in the 'SubString Search' it retrieves all of the different types of leukaemia. 'Searching for an Exact Match'does precisely that, although it does not worry about upper and lower case; 'All Fragments' will look for all the parts of your word in any order; and 'Any Fragment' will look for any part of your word. It is not always essential to use MeSH, but it is advisable to optimise searching, but some journals insist on MeSH terms for keywords (see Chap. 3). You might find the MeSH on Demand or MeSH Browswer helpful here [7]. Some journals also feature a 'highlights' or 'what this study adds' section; these are usually in the form of bullet points. Whether or not these are required, you should be thinking about how to summarise your review into a clear and meaningful message.

While journals differ in presentation, there is increasing standardisation on the scientific criteria for a systematic review. The Preferred Reporting Items for Systematic Reviews and Meta-Analyses (PRISMA) guidelines [8] are endorsed by most scientific journals in healthcare. Reviewers must comply with the 27 items on the PRISMA checklist, and some journals require this to be submitted alongside the manuscript. This is shown in Table 11.1.

An important point to remember is that PRISMA is a reporting checklist, not a quality assessment tool; it only tells you what should be in your review.

Reporting guidelines have also been produced specifically for qualitative research. An example is the enhancing transparency in reporting the synthesis of qualitative research (ENTREQ) tool [9] which is now established as a reporting guideline for qualitative literature reviews. Its 21 items are shown in Table 11.2.

11.3   Choosing a Journal

If you are submitting your review for publication, take care to choose an appropriate journal. This may be decided at the outset, or perhaps at a later stage, when the findings have emerged. In Chap. 1, we described trends in academic literature, with a proliferation of journals and a steady shift towards open access. Wherever there is money to be made, unscrupulous opportunists try to exploit the naïve. In the publishing world, this problem manifests in 'predatory journals'. For the uninitiated, these are journals that exist primarily for the purpose of extracting money from unsuspecting authors, who might think that any journal with an apparently authoritative name

Table 11.1 PRISMA checklist items

Number	Domain	Item	Detail (abridged)
1	Title		Identify as systematic review and/or meta-analysis
2	Abstract		Structured summary
3	Introduction	Rationale	In context of existing knowledge
4		Objectives	How review question was answered
5	Method	Protocol	Indicate if and where review was registered
6		Eligibility criteria	Clearly specified, with justification
7		Information sources	Databases and other sources specified
8		Search strategy	Search terms and process described
9		Screening	Process described
10		Data extraction	How data were sought
11		Data items	Variables included
12		Risk of bias within studies	How risk was assessed
13		Summary measures	Outcome of review (e.g. risk ratio, mean difference)
14		Synthesis of results	How data were synthesised
15		Risk of bias across studies	How overall risk was assessed
16		Additional analyses	(e.g. sensitivity or subgroup analyses)
17	Results	Study selection	Number screened and eligible
18		Study characteristics	Summary of eligible studies
19		Risk of bias within studies	Findings of bias assessment
20		Results of studies	Relevant results shown for each study
21		Synthesis of results	Results of meta-analysis/synthesis
22		Risk of bias across studies	Findings of overall bias assessment
23		Additional analyses	(e.g. results of sensitivity or subgroup analyses)
24	Discussion	Summary of results	Clear summary of review outcomes
25		Limitations	Critical appraisal of strengths and weaknesses
26		Conclusions	Implications/recommendations
27	Funding		Sources of funding stated

must be legitimate. Publication is often agreed immediately, with little evidence of peer review and none of the normal quality control such as proofreading. Your paper will not be read very much, because it won't appear in research databases and possibly not Google Scholar either.

Jeffrey Beall, a librarian at the University of Colorado, created and maintained a list of predatory journals. This became known as Beall's List. In some cases, the named and shamed publishers threatened defamation lawsuits, and eventually Beall terminated the list, although archived versions can still be found by Internet search [10]; if you perform a search for 'predatory journals list' you may find newer lists. It should be said that this list was always controversial, with some arguing that this approach shows a lack of understanding of open access journals, which operate differently in many ways to traditional format journals, most notably by charging authors a fee for publication. Our advice is to ask subject experts

Table 11.2 ENTREQ checklist items

Number	Item	Guidance
1	Aim	Present the question to be answered by the synthesis
2	Synthesis methodology	State the method of synthesis and justify its application
3	Approach to searching	Show whether search was a priori or iterative
4	Inclusion criteria	Specify inclusion and exclusion criteria
5	Data sources	Describe and justify data sources
6	Electronic search strategy	Describe literature search
7	Study screening methods	Describe screening process
8	Study characteristics	Show number of studies screened and explain exclusions
9	Study selection results	Summarise design and publication details of included studies
10	Rationale for appraisal	Describe process and rationale for study appraisal
11	Appraisal items	State tools, framework and criteria for study appraisal
12	Appraisal process	Indicate whether study appraisal was conducted by one or more reviewer and whether consensus was achieved
13	Appraisal results	Present results of study appraisal and indicate any weighting of studies
14	Data extraction	Show which parts of studies and their data were analysed
15	Software	State any application used in coding and analysis
16	Number of reviewers	Identify who was involved ion coding and analysis
17	Coding	Describe process of coding study data
18	Study comparison	Describe how comparisons were made between and within studies
19	Derivation of themes	Explain whether themes/constructs were discerned deductively or inductively
20	Quotations	Provide quotations from studies to illustrate themes/constructs
21	Synthesis output	Findings of the synthesis should present a new interpretation rather than merely a summary of the studies

in your area if you are not sure about a journal. As soon as your publication paper published, you will begin to receive emails from predatory journals. Genuine academic journals do not normally seek business in this way unless you are really considered to be an expert, in which case you may be invited to submit a paper to a special edition or write an editorial. These predatory invitations are often riddled with academic error, with a grandiose address: you may be promoted to 'professor', with a message like this:

Dear esteemed Professor XXXX. We read your fascinating and informative paper on XXXX, and we would be loving to receive your expert articles for *International Journal of XYZ* [often in no way related to the subject of the paper you wrote] Your researches will be feature in the next edition.

Unscrupulous, dubious—this applies to conferences too. Journal editors and conference organisers solicit for articles and speakers and will usually publish an edition or run a conference if they get enough takers, but the quality may not be very good. Such publication or presentation will not enhance your profile and could reduce your credibility.

Having warned of the journals to avoid, let us now consider the fully fledged academic publication outlets. Whatever the merits of this, some journals are considered to be of higher standing than others, although exactly what is meant by this is not always clear. The established measure is the journal impact factor. This is a score based on how often (on average) a paper in the journal is cited in a given time period; therefore it is the ratio of citations to the number of papers published in the journal. One of the most widely used impact factors is Journal Citation Reports [11], which measures over a rolling 2-year period. Generic or multidisciplinary journals generally have higher scores than specialist journals simply because they are read by more people.

Impact factor is not the only consideration in selecting a journal, although for most authors it is important, and you will often find the latest figure on the journal's website. A novice author will usually aim low, as submitting to a highly competitive leading journal in the field may have minimal prospects of success, and delay publication due to rejection and the need to resume the process with another journal. Editors will not send a manuscript for peer review if it does not fit the standards and scope of the journal, and if submitting to a well-resourced journal, a paper that is incorrectly formatted or referenced may be immediately returned by the editorial office for appropriate changes to be made. If a manuscript is reviewed and rejected, at least the author will get useful advice on improving the work, boosting the chance of publication with another journal. Authors may have a hierarchy of journals in mind. So you may first try the *International Journal of Elation* (impact factor 5); if rejected, you may then send to the *Journal of Happiness* (impact factor 2), and if not accepted there either, you may resort to the *Journal of Mild Satisfaction* (impact factor 0.5). You will find this process much easier if you use reference management software as this will do the job of changing the references for you. Reformatting a long list of references really is the dullest job.

11.4 Writing Style

Academic literature is perceived to be dry and formulaic, with little leeway for lyrical flourish. Scientific journals ensure that papers fit a template, are written in the language of the discipline and do not exceed tight word limits. Journals publishing qualitative work allow more creativity, but house style and reporting requirements apply there too. However, there is no rule against good writing!

Your paper should tell a story, and tell it well. To be truthful, most research papers are not fully read, as students, scholars or practitioners may only be interested in the method, results or conclusion sections. The opening paragraph is vital in luring readers beyond the abstract and to read the paper from beginning to end. Writing of high quality is enjoyable to read, whatever the complexity of the topic. For those who struggle with academic writing, we suggest the Manchester Academic Phrasebank for examples of critical, defining, describing and other phrases that may be useful http://www.phrasebank.manchester.ac.uk/.

One way of making your report appear interesting is to use an analogy or metaphor. We used a historical connection in the introduction to our systematic review of social media and mental health in younger people [12]:

> New technology can transform society, but fears have been raised about its physical, social and psychological consequences. This has historical precedent. In the nineteenth century, many people were diagnosed with 'railway sickness', a condition attributed to the unnatural motions of train travel, most frequently observed in passengers who had faced backwards.

There was no direct scientific importance in alluding to an unrelated paper in the *Lancet* from 1895, but our likening of past to present health scares was thought-provoking, emphasising the need for critical thinking. Just as railway sickness was unfounded, is there a moral panic about the Internet? This suggests that the writer is trying to engage the reader on a higher level than simply relaying the process and outcome of a research exercise.

11.5 Disseminate Widely

Presenting to academic or clinical audiences is one way of reporting your work beyond the journal readership. This may be within your organisation or at a conference. While presenting at conferences is fundamental to an academic career, the amount of people that you will reach may not be high. If your publication profile is at an early stage of development, you may be granted a poster presentation, which gives you the opportunity to discuss your work with other researchers and to engage in networking. Sometimes you are given a short 3–5 min presentation 'slot' alongside this, and you may like to take smaller copies of your poster for people to take away. Your work may be chosen for a spoken presentation. Esteemed professors speak at plenary sessions, but the majority of 'lesser mortals' are given seminar slots of about 15 min, with the delegates choosing between your talk and perhaps five other parallel seminars. However, your abstract will be published in the conference proceedings, which may be collated by research databases.

A quicker and further reaching means of dissemination is to draw attention of the newspapers or other mass media. If you are in a university, consult the communications/public relations officer, who will have expertise in detecting whether you have a message of public interest, and how to frame your findings for a particular readership. A press release may be issued. This should be sharpened to a fine point: health editors are bombarded with researchers seeking publicity for their work. Greenhalgh [13] observed that researchers often fail in their attempts to communicate with the media:

> Some of the worst literature I have ever read in my life consists of so-called press releases written by academics…Researchers often make a boring study even more boring when they try to popularise it.

Numerous websites publish short articles by researchers, making findings more widely available than the full report in an academic journal. Typically the maximum length is 800 words and gives you practice in writing succinctly and for a wider audience. Use lay language and avoid acronyms, technical or theoretical terminology or statistical formulae. Journals such as the *Nursing Times* publish readers' blogs (www.nursingtimes.net). Other websites may be found online (e.g. https://nurse.org/articles/top-50-fantastic-blogs-for-nurses). The Conversation (www.the-conversation.com) is a reputable website for scholarly research and commentary; authors must have a doctorate. Don't try to cram all your findings into a short article. Minimise use of hyperlinks: they are distracting and sometimes the redirected reader won't return to your piece. There are limitless opportunities for self-publishing, as in a personal blog, although readers may be confined to your followers and friends. Every channel should be considered, however, as a means of increasing exposure.

Twitter is useful to disseminate your article (if open access), simply by posting the link. A short message preceding the link will tell your followers why your review is important. You should also tweet any other articles you have written on the review, as above. Everybody starts with a small number of followers, but this grows steadily if you follow others and tweet regularly. Twitter enables you to respond to anyone's tweets, and you could find yourself exchanging messages with leading figures in your field. Use hashtags to get involved in Twitter discussions relating to your topic.

Another good way of disseminating your work is by registering on ResearchGate, a website that may be described as Facebook for researchers. ResearchGate allows you to present your publication profile and current research activity to a vast number of users. You can use ResearchGate to send communicate with other researchers in your field. Copies of your papers may be loaded, but check first that you have permission from the journal (this will not be a problem if you have paid for open access). Otherwise, you could be infringing copyright law. By placing the abstract on ResearchGate, you are publicising your work legally, and other people can contact you for further information (if requested, you may send a copy of your paper by e-mail).

Institutional repositories are of great value. Most universities make copies of research by staff and students freely available. You should definitely contact your university librarian or repository coordinator to find out about this, as there may be sanctions for not depositing your work in a repository (it is also bad science not to do so). Your activity and publications should also be shown on department or faculty websites, wherever possible. Universities and healthcare organisations are large communities, and there may be numerous members who would be interested in your work. Instead of staying in silos, researchers in such communities should be nurturing interdisciplinary and interdepartmental relations, potentially leading to fruitful partnerships. Information on your research should be publicly available online, so that people outside can read about your projects and outputs; it is vital to update this information regularly.

Open access, once considered a nicety, is now becoming a requirement. In the UK, for papers to be considered for the Research Excellence Framework, the final accepted version must be deposited in an institutional repository, a repository service shared between multiple institutions, or a subject repository within 3 months of acceptance (i.e. the date you receive acceptance for publication) [14], while in the USA, all National Institutes of Health (NIH)-funded researchers have to submit the final peer-reviewed journal manuscripts to PubMed Central immediately upon acceptance [15]. Note that these are not the publishers' formatted versions over which the publishers retain copyright (unless you have paid for open access). If you want a paper and can't get it via your library, there are various places where papers are deposited, so it is always worth doing a search-engine search for titles.

11.6   Measuring Impact

A systematic review should inform practice, but it is not always clear how much influence findings and recommendations have on practitioners and patients. Sometimes new evidence takes a while to reach the clinical setting. A starting point for measuring impact is how much your review is being read. Some journals show the amount of downloads for each paper, on the website. You can also estimate the level of interest from activity data on ResearchGate. If you have written about your review on a website there may be a 'hit' count. *The Conversation* website provides authors with detailed metrics on reads, tweets and shares, including a pie chart of where your article is read. Twitter data show the level of engagement with each tweet.

The old adage of 'publish or perish' is a brutal truth for anyone embarking on an academic career: nobody can rest on their laurels after one successful project. However, possibly more important to researchers than the number of published papers is the frequency of citation. As soon as your paper appears, it could be included in the background or literature review in another writer's paper, which will enhance the prospects of further referencing. Each published paper is like a snowball, gradually gathering citations. The count in Google Scholar includes citations not only in journal but also postgraduate academic assignments (dissertations and theses). As academic employees know, universities tend not to use Google Scholar for citation data, but a scientific database such as Scopus or Web of Science that restricts citations to peer-reviewed literature, with limited inclusion of journals of very low impact factor. One should be careful about citations as a measure of impact; however, the number of citations depends on the status of the discipline or specialty as well as the importance of your paper. A paper on a promising new treatment for 'obscuritis' published in the world leading *Journal of Obscurity* will reach a narrower audience than a paper with insignificant findings on a common condition in a widely read journal. Methodological papers of cross-specialty relevance are often highly cited.

Coverage of journals by research databases has considerable effect on the writer's impact rating, which is known as the '*h* index'. Physicist Hirsch [16] at the University of California, San Diego, devised this index to estimate 'the importance, significance, and broad impact of a scientist's cumulative research contributions'. It is a score determined by the number of your papers for which you have at least the same number of citations. So, if you have had four papers published and two have been cited twice each, your *h* index is 2. To get to 3, you need both of those papers to be cited again, plus another of your papers to get three citations. The *h* index is generally accepted as a firm but fair measure, but not perfect (e.g. it might work against a woman whose surname changes on marriage, although this can be resolved). You can look up colleagues' or rivals' scores in Scopus or Web of Science to compare your progress!

11.7 Review of Reviews

Having completed your review, you may be interested in comparing your results with those of others who have also done reviews. This may be an informal comparison, or you may want to do this formally. A review of reviews is known as an 'umbrella review', and like every other types of review, there are methods for undertaking this. In principle, an umbrella review is no different to any other types of systematic review, except that the raw material is reviews rather than original studies. The results can be presented graphically in the form of a forest plot or in tabular form if this is not appropriate or possible. Each review needs to be critically appraised using the appropriate tool, for example, AMSTAR [17] and ROBIS [18] as described earlier, just as you would if using individual studies [19]. One important fact to remember is that the reviews included will almost certainly be using the same studies, so each review is not providing independent results. It is analogous to primary study using the same sample. Because of this, it is not really appropriate to pool the results. What may be more illuminating might be the case where there are different reviews looking a slightly different aspects of the same question, for example, how well a drug works? and how do patients feel about it?

11.8 Is There a Replication Crisis?

A major controversy that has arisen in scientific research is the replication or replicability crisis. This refers to the difficulty that is often experienced in repeating the results of an original study or indeed a systematic review. Some variation in results is to be expected due to random differences in study participants or differences in the setting, personnel or equipment. However, the results should not be so different that the evidence is unreliable. Probably the two most serious replication issues are when the direction of the result differs, for example, thinking a treatment works when it may actually make a condition worse; or when a Type I or Type II statistical error is made (see Chap. 6) because these may actually affect patient care. Because systematic reviews are considered to be a high level of evidence and so can be very influential, it is particularly important that these are replicable. Different people asking the same question should find the same papers and get the same results.

There are many possible detractors from replicability, for example, dubious research practices such as omitting data points or failing to publish contradictory results [20]. Problems with replicability have been found in one of the most prestigious science journals in the world, *Science* and *Nature* [21]. A stark demonstration of the replication problem was a study in which 29 research teams were sent the same data set for analysis. The teams each attempted to answer the research question of whether football (soccer) referees are more likely to give red cards to dark-skin-toned players than to light-skin-toned players. Their results varied widely, with 21 combinations of covariates produced from the dataset. Twenty teams found a statistically significant relationship while nine did not, and the odds ratios varied from 0.89 to 2.93. However, there were 11 teams with similar findings, their odds ratios varying from 1.28 to 1.48 and all being statistically significant [22].

Another fact of life is that people, journal editors included, like to find 'new' things. Thus there may be a premium on novelty, and you are unlikely to get a paper published which replicates previous findings however worthy an endeavour this might be scientifically. Most people know that Neil Armstrong was the first man on the Moon, but fewer remember Buzz Aldrin who was the second. Can you remember who the third was? This is not necessarily a reflection of the scientific work that they did on the moon; it is just that we tend to remember the first. Perhaps more worryingly, once something has been shown 'to work any incentive to continue questioning, this may be lost. Replicating research findings is of the upmost importance scientifically if not reputationally. Refuting previous findings may be even more important.

Another reason for replication problems may be a practice that researchers do without really realising it. It is known under a number of terms including P-hacking, data-dredging, snooping, fishing, significance-chasing and double-dipping. These all refer to the process of trying multiple tests or analyses until you get the result that you want, for example, getting that p-value of 0.051 down to 0.049 and so being able to report it as 'statistically significant'. These are then the results that you report. One at least partial solution to this is to de-emphasise p-values, another may be preregistration of analysis plans, although rigidly sticking to a plan may hinder researchers who do see new patterns in datasets and a more complex two-stage system of 'preregistered replication' has been suggested. This could consist of smaller exploratory studies followed by a larger confirmatory study [23]. As ever, probably the best defence against this is transparency, for example, publication of data sets and analysis plans allows for others to replicate analyses. If you have taken our advice to use the computer programme R (or a similar programme) to do your analysis, you should also publish your full code.

11.9   Conclusion

What's next? If you are a healthcare practitioner, first and foremost, you may have opportunity to put your recommendations into practice. You will also have issued recommendations for research. Perhaps your review was a precursor to further study at Master's or PhD level. You may have set the scene for a study proposal and a funding application. If you have done your review well, confirmed by a high academic mark or publication in a reputable journal, you have knowledge and experience to impart to others. As we hope to have shown with this book, the right way to do a systematic review is not convoluted but an exhibition of logic. As a final thought, throughout this book we have emphasised best practice and the need for transparency. Be honest and explicit about what you have done. And expect that transparency in any other reviews that you read. As a consumer of research, be sceptical. Always.

References

1. Research Excellence Framework (2014) Impact Case Studies. https://impact.ref.ac.uk/casestudies/FAQ.aspx. Accessed 6 Mar 2020.
2. UK Research & Innovation (2018) Excellence with impact—UK Research and Innovation. https://www.ukri.org/innovation/excellence-with-impact/. Accessed 6 Mar 2020
3. Munthe-Kaas H, Nøkleby H, Lewin S, Glenton C (2020) The TRANSFER approach for assessing the transferability of systematic review findings. BMC Med Res Methodol 20:11. https://doi.org/10.1186/s12874-019-0834-5
4. Schünemann H, Brożek J, Guyatt G, Oxman A (2013) GRADE handbook. https://gdt.gradepro.org/app/handbook/handbook.html. Accessed 6 Mar 2020
5. Lewin S, Booth A, Glenton C et al (2018) Applying GRADE-CERQual to qualitative evidence synthesis findings: introduction to the series. Implement Sci 13:2. https://doi.org/10.1186/s13012-017-0688-3
6. Committee on Publication Ethics (2019) COPE discussion document: authorship. https://publicationethics.org/node/34946. Accessed 11 Mar 2020
7. National Library of Medicine (2018) Suggestions for finding author keywords using MeSH Tools. https://www.nlm.nih.gov/mesh/authors.html. Accessed 6 Mar 2020
8. Moher D, Liberati A, Tetzlaff J et al (2009) Preferred reporting items for systematic reviews and meta-analyses: the PRISMA statement. PLoS Med 6:e1000097. https://doi.org/10.1371/journal.pmed.1000097
9. Tong A, Flemming K, McInnes E et al (2012) Enhancing transparency in reporting the synthesis of qualitative research: ENTREQ. BMC Med Res Methodol 12:181. https://doi.org/10.1186/1471-2288-12-181
10. Beall J (2017). Beallslist.net—Beall's list of predatory journals and publishers. https://beallslist.weebly.com/. Accessed 6 Mar 2020
11. Clarivate Analytics (2018) The clarivate analytics impact factor. In: Web of Science Group. https://clarivate.com/webofsciencegroup/essays/impact-factor/. Accessed 6 Mar 2020
12. McCrae N, Gettings S, Purssell E (2017) Social media and depressive symptoms in childhood and adolescence: a systematic review. Adolesc Res Rev 2:315–330. https://doi.org/10.1007/s40894-017-0053-4
13. Greenhalgh T (2018) How to implement evidence-based healthcare. Wiley, Hoboken, NJ
14. Research Excellence Framework (2019) REF 2021: overview of open access policy and guidance. https://www.ref.ac.uk/media/1228/open_access_summary__v1_0.pdf. Accessed 17 Apr 2020
15. National Institutes of Health (2014) When and how to comply. https://publicaccess.nih.gov/. Accessed 6 Mar 2020
16. Hirsch JE (2005) An index to quantify an individual's scientific research output. Proc Natl Acad Sci 102:16569–16572. https://doi.org/10.1073/pnas.0507655102
17. Shea BJ, Reeves BC, Wells G et al (2017) AMSTAR 2: a critical appraisal tool for systematic reviews that include randomised or non-randomised studies of healthcare interventions, or both. BMJ 358:j4008. https://doi.org/10.1136/bmj.j4008
18. Whiting P, Savović J, Higgins JPT et al (2016) ROBIS: a new tool to assess risk of bias in systematic reviews was developed. J Clin Epidemiol 69:225–234. https://doi.org/10.1016/j.jclinepi.2015.06.005

19. Aromataris E, Fernandez R, Godfrey CM et al (2015) Summarizing systematic reviews: methodological development, conduct and reporting of an umbrella review approach. Int J Evid Based Healthc 13:132–140. https://doi.org/10.1097/XEB.0000000000000055
20. Fanelli D (2018) Opinion: is science really facing a reproducibility crisis, and do we need it to? Proc Natl Acad Sci U S A 115:2628–2631. https://doi.org/10.1073/pnas.1708272114
21. Camerer CF, Dreber A, Holzmeister F et al (2018) Evaluating the replicability of social science experiments in Nature and Science between 2010 and 2015. Nat Hum Behav 2:637–644. https://doi.org/10.1038/s41562-018-0399-z
22. Silberzahn R, Uhlmann EL, Martin DP et al (2018) Many analysts, one data set: making transparent how variations in analytic choices affect results. Adv Methods Pract Psychol Sci 1:337–356. https://doi.org/10.1177/2515245917747646
23. Nuzzo R (2014) Scientific method: statistical errors. Nature 506:150–152. https://doi.org/10.1038/506150a

Appendix A: Using WebPlotDigitizer

Sometimes you have a figure and it is not necessarily easy to extract numbers from it. For this you need an application such as the WebPlotDigitizer. This can be accessed here: https://apps.automeris.io/wpd/.

This programme is distributed under the GNU Affero General Public License Version 3.

When you open it, you get a screen that looks like this:

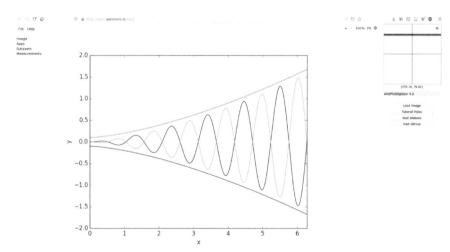

You then need to save the graphic and import it through the Load Image button on the right-hand side. You then navigate to the figure that you want to upload; you should have previously saved it as a graphical file. This will then appear in the window in the application.

Here you can see an example from a paper looking at Pneumococcal carriage among children under five in Accra, Ghana; five years after the introduction of pneumococcal conjugate vaccine, this particular figure shows antibiotic resistance against different serotypes of pneumococcus (Dayie et al. 2019). We are going to look at the bottom figure in detail here.

© The Editor(s) (if applicable) and The Author(s), under exclusive license to Springer Nature Switzerland AG 2020
E. Purssell, N. McCrae, *How to Perform a Systematic Literature Review*,
https://doi.org/10.1007/978-3-030-49672-2

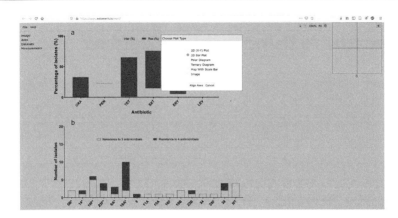

After which you choose the plot type—in this case a 2D Bar Plot. You then need to click on Align Axis so that it knows the scale used for the bars.

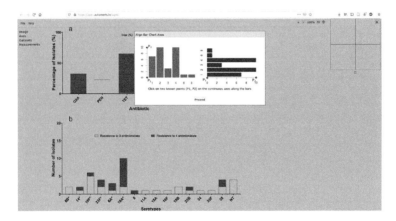

In this case, the scale is on the *y*-axis, so you click the top and bottom of the axis and give the application the range, which is figure (a) above is 0–100 and in (b) 0–20.

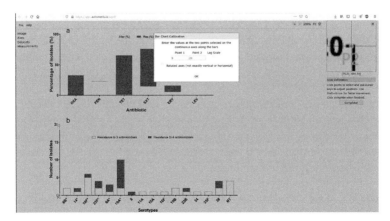

If you look at the top left-hand size, you can see an expanded view of Point 2 to help you do this accurately. Point 1 is at 0 and Point 2 is at 20. You then click on each bar to see how far up the *y*-axis each extends.

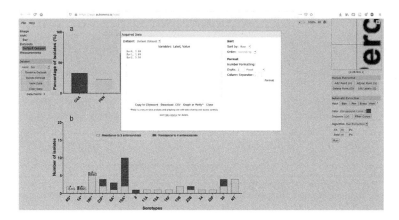

Here you can see that we had a look at the first three bars, and then pressed View Data to see the actual number associated with each bar. There are multiple options to export the data as a .csv file or via the clipboard. You can also change the number of figures after the decimal point.

References

Dayie NTKD, Tettey EY, Newman MJ et al (2019) Pneumococcal carriage among children under five in Accra, Ghana, five years after the introduction of pneumococcal conjugate vaccine. BMC Pediatr 19:316. https://doi.org/10.1186/s12887-019-1690-5

Rohatgi A (2020) WebPlotDigitizer - Extract data from plots, images, and maps. https://automeris.io/WebPlotDigitizer/. Accessed 16 Jul 2020

Appendix B:
How to Do a Meta-analysis Using R

How to Do a Meta-analysis in R

This chapter is going to show you how to undertake a meta-analysis using a package called meta (with a little 'm') in a programme called R (big R). The good news is that all of the materials that you need for this are freely available; the not so good news is that R takes a bit of getting used to. However, when you have got used to it you will find it among your best academic friends as it has so many useful packages that do so many useful things, not just meta-analysis but advanced graphics, general statistics, data mining, qualitative analysis, spatial analysis, survey analysis….the list is virtually endless.

Installing R

To install R, go to the R homepage https://cran.r-project.org/ where you will find instructions for installing R on Linux, Mac and Windows.

If you are using Linux, you will find the interface is dreadful, as it uses the Terminal, and even if you are using the other operating systems you may still prefer a nicer interface than you get with R on its own. There are a few of these, but the most commonly used and the one that you will normally see on YouTube videos is called R Studio https://rstudio.com/ (look for the free version). Other options are: rkward https://rkward.kde.org/, Tinn-R https://sourceforge.net/projects/tinn-r/ or Rattle https://sourceforge.net/projects/tinn-r/

Depending upon which you go for: plain R or one of the other options when you open the programme up, you will get a fairly blank screen and a cursor. Although you may find some buttons and menus, R is really at its best when you type code in the form of a script rather than using buttons and menus. There are two reasons for this; firstly, it means that your work is 100% replicable, and secondly it means that if you have a problem you can send your code to your supervisor/second author/significant other and publish it with your paper making your work super-transparent.

© The Editor(s) (if applicable) and The Author(s), under exclusive license to Springer Nature Switzerland AG 2020
E. Purssell, N. McCrae, *How to Perform a Systematic Literature Review*,
https://doi.org/10.1007/978-3-030-49672-2

Packages

R does have some built-in capabilities; it can do *t*-tests, ANOVA and all those sorts of things from scratch in what we call 'base-R'. If you have downloaded R, that is what you currently have. In order to do most of the many, many things that R can do, you need to download different packages. There are, at the time of writing, 15,359 different packages of which a number has the capability to do meta-analysis. You can see the full range of meta-analysis packages here https://cran.r-project.org/web/views/MetaAnalysis.html. We are going to use one of these, a package called **meta** which has its own homepage here https://CRAN.R-project.org/package=meta. One of the links on that page leads to the **meta Reference manual** which you should have a look at, but if it looks like gobbledygook don't worry, this chapter is here to guide you through it.

Start R

Start R by clicking on the appropriate icon; this will be the blue R if you are using Base R or the appropriate icon if you are using a different interface.

The first thing to do is to download the packages that you want. You do this by clicking the

Packages menu, then the **Install packages** option. Then scroll down until you find meta and click on it. You will be asked where you would like to download it from, choose somewhere near (or nice) and you should then see all sorts of things happening, don't worry about it let it all happen.

What You Will See

If you are using Base R, you will start by seeing one single window, this is called the **Console** and it is where the results of your analysis will appear. Resist the temptation to type code here as it will not be saved. To type your code, you need the **Text editor** by going to File then New script and you then see a new box appear. This is the Text editor where you will type your code and from which your code can be saved for future use. It is most important that this is where you type your code from now on. If you are using R Studio, you will see four boxes when you first open the programme; your **Text editor** is on the top left and your **Console** on the bottom left.

Things to Know About R

1. It is free, free as in completely free. For this, we should thank the countless people who wrote and maintain R and all of the packages that are available.
2. It runs on all major platforms, but the details vary. At work, I use Windows which has control and R as the method of running functions; it is different for Macs and different again for Linux which I use at home. One of the reasons for

using programmes such as R Studio and the other options listed at the start is that they are the same across all platforms, you just highlight the code you want and press run.

3. R does what you tell it to and no more. If you tell it to do a meta-analysis, it will; but it will not print the results unless you ask it to. You can get the results by just typing in the name of your meta-analysis.

4. In the spirit of doing what you ask and no more, even though you have downloaded a package it will not actually run unless you tell R to run it. The function for this is library(name of package). I think of this as being like going to a library to take out my favourite book (or package). If you think about it that this makes sense, you might easily have 100 packages downloaded; it would be very wasteful of your computer's resources to have them all running all of the time.

5. While on the subject of running packages, some packages rely on other packages to run. So meta uses metafor for example. This is known as a dependency. You need not worry about it as generally R knows what is dependent on what and will look after it.

6. R is case sensitive, so Ed is not the same as ed. Note that meta has a little 'm', as does metafor which your computer will try and turn into the word metaphor when you put it in reports, while MAd has a capital 'M' and a 'D'.

7. The most common errors in my experience are capitalisation errors (see above), missing " " around file locations or text arguments, and spelling errors.

8. You can annotate your code with #. R ignores everything after the # until you get to a new line. So you could write funnel(MetaB) #this is my funnel plot! and R will do the plot and ignore the comment. You can write notes to remind yourself or perhaps most importantly for other people when reading your code about what things mean or why you did them.

9. If you have a very long line of code, you can split it over two or more lines. R will just go on reading the function until it gets to the end. It will know it is at the end when it can do something, often this will be the final close bracket. If you see a + in the Console, it means that R is waiting for something to complete the function, it is often a closing bracket.

10. R error messages are not intuitive. Let Google be your friend here!

11. There is a large and active R community who are very helpful, but they will expect that you have done a little research yourself first.

12. There are loads and loads of online resources. For meta-analysis, I suggest the manuals of the packages used; the metafor manual is long but very helpful, and this online book is very good:
    Harrer MH, Cuijpers PDP, Furukawa PDTA, Ebert DD (2019). Doing meta-analysis in R. Retrieved from https://bookdown.org/MathiasHarrer/ Doing_Meta_Analysis_in_R/

13. Always save your code. Don't worry about saving anything else as long as you have saved your code. It will be saved with a .R file name. You can share your code either by sending the .R file to your supervisor, or by opening it with an external Text editor.

Starting Meta

Although you have downloaded meta onto your machine, you can't use it until you run it in this session. Click on the **Text editor** so it is active and type the words: `library(meta)`

If you are using Base R, then highlight these words and press control and R together; if you are using R Studio, just type into the box on the top left-hand side then press Run. If you are using a Mac or Linux the keystrokes to run the command may be slightly different.

We are going to try to answer the question 'does coffee make you brainy?' Having read everything that you have, you may think there are some limitations to this question but just go with us for the moment, you can critique this question later. Having done a full search of the literature, we found four papers that had data to answer this question. They are:

Hogervorst et al. (1998)
Delayed recall (young)
caffeine mean = 10.6 (1.5), $n = 10$; placebo mean = 11.3 (1.8), $n = 10$
Twenty minutes after completion of the fifth trial, subjects were asked to recall as many of the previously learned words as possible that were presented visually (delayed recall or long-term memory).

Mednick et al. (2008)
Recall at 20 min
caffeine mean = 12.25 (3.5), $n = 12$; placebo mean = 13.70 (3.0), $n = 11$
Recall of Word List 1 at 20 min

Ryan et al. (2002)
Long-delay free recall (Morning)
caffeine mean = 11.8 (2.9), $n = 20$; decaffeinated mean = 11 (2.7), $n = 20$
Long-delay free recall (Afternoon)
caffeine mean = 11.7 (2.8), $n = 20$; decaffeinated mean = 8.9 (3), $n = 20$
A 20-min delay occurs next, followed by both free recall of the original list (long-delay free recall)

Sherman et al. (2016)
Cued recall task
caffeine mean = 0.44 (0.13), $n = 30$; decaffeinated mean = 0.34 (0.13), $n = 30$
The explicit word-stem cued recall task followed immediately.

If you look at these numbers, without going into too many details of the papers you can see just from these numbers that they are clearly using different scales. If you were confident, you might decide to convert them to the same scale, but you may not be sufficiently confident to do this or you may not be able to do this—the scales may not be comparable at all.

Now put these numbers into a spreadsheet that looks something like this:

Study	Mcaff	SDcaff	Ncaff	Mdecaff	SDdecaff	Ndecaff
Hogervorst et al. (1998)	10.6	1.5	10	11.3	1.8	10
Mednick et al. (2008)	12.25	3.5	12	13.7	3	11
Ryan et al. (2002)	11.3	3.4	20	9.2	2.3	20
Sherman et al. (2016)	0.44	0.13	30	0.34	0.13	30

and then save it as a .csv file. Do this by selecting save as and then choosing csv rather than the default option that your spreadsheet programme provides you with. You may find that your software automatically changes SDcaff to Sdcaff. This is not important, either suppress this feature, or just change SD into Sd in all of the commands that follow.

Now comes probably the most tricky bit, that is getting these data into R. There are other ways, but the method I prefer is to use code rather than buttons and menus (remember this makes your code totally reproducible and transparent).

To find the location of your file, type this into the Text editor:

```
file.choose()
```

and then press control and R together, when the dialogue box comes up, find your file and open it. This will not actually open your file, but it will make R display its location in the **Console**.

Now go back to your Text editor and type:

```
Dat<-read.csv("XXXX", header = TRUE)
```

where XXXXX.csv is the location of your file that you just copied. Then press control and R together. You should see your function appear in red in the Console and nothing else; if so, well done it has worked; if you get an error, there are two common reasons for this. The first is that you have not copied the location from 'to'—it must include both; the second is that if you are copying and pasting the functions from here, try retyping the " " as sometimes this changes when you copy from text in different fonts.

Let us quickly have a look at what we did here. R works by creating things called objects. The command that creates an object is the less than sign and the hyphen <- to make a backwards arrow. I chose to call this Dat, but you can call it pretty much anything you like.

It says 'do the thing on the right and then call it the thing on the left', so in this case we are telling R to read a.csv file read.csv in the location "XXXX.csv" that you copied in. The header=TRUE argument is telling R that the first row in your spreadsheet contains column headings and not data. Note that TRUE is in capitals, this is important.

The next thing to do is to have a look at what data you have imported. To do this, simply type the name of our object into the Console. Can you work out what you need to type? It is the name allocated to your data, in this case Dat.

Now we are going to get ready to do the meta-analysis. First, we need to run the **meta** package by typing:

```
library(meta)
```

and then undertake the meta-analysis using the metacont function from the **meta** package. If you have a look at the manual, you will see it described thus: 'Calculation of fixed and random effects estimates for meta-analyses with continuous outcome data'. Now look further down and you will see the slightly scary looking section entitled **Usage** which shows the arguments that are used with this function. There are a lot of them; the good news is that you don't need to use most of them as they have default values:

```
metacont(
n.e,
mean.e,
sd.e,
n.c,
mean.c,
sd.c,
studlab,
data = NULL
sm
```

So we have the `metacont` function followed by n.e= after which we type the name of the column in which the numbers in the experimental group is to be found, so in this case it would be `n.e=Ncaff`, then `mean.e=Mcaff` for the mean in the experimental group, and `sd.e=SDcaff` for the standard deviation in the experimental group. We then do the same for the control group like this `n.c=Ndecaff`, `mean.c=Mdecaff` and `sd.c=SDdecaff`. Remember if your software has converted `SDcaff` in to `Sdcaff`, you will need to make the appropriate changes to this and `SDdecaff`.

The next thing that we need to do is to tell R where the study labels are; we will need this for the forest plot to label the different studies, the argument for this is `studlab`. If you look at the data again, you will see that these labels are in a column called `Study`, so type `studlab=Study`.

Now we need to tell R what effect measure we want for our meta-analysis. If all our studies use the same measure, we can simply use the mean difference, the mean in the experimental group minus the mean in the control group; but in this case, we can't do that because they have used different scales. So instead of using "MD" which means mean difference, we use "SMD" or standardised mean difference. If you can't remember what this means, please refer to Chap. 7.

Finally, we have told R which columns to look for and what to do, but not where these columns are. They are of course in our data which we imported called `MetaA`. This goes after the data argument like this `data=Dat`

This gives a final line of code that looks like this:

```
MetaA<-metacont(n.e=Ncaff, mean.e=Mcaff, sd.e=SDcaff,
n.c=Ndecaff, mean.c=Mdecaff, sd.c=SDdecaff, studlab=Study,
sm="SMD", data=Dat)
```

Hopefully you will recognise the <- which means that when you did the meta-analysis you gave it a name, in this case the very imaginative `MetaB`; don't give it the same name as your data as it will overwrite the data.

If you highlight the whole line of code, then as before press `control` and R together, and if it is correct the function should ping over to the **Console** as before with no error message. You will notice that it does not actually display your result;

however, to do this go to the **Console** and type in the name of our meta-analysis (which is `MetaB`).

You will probably want to produce a forest plot (who doesn't!?!) The function for this is `forest`.

Have a look at the manual and you will see:

```
forest(
x,
test.overall.fixed,
test.overall.random
```

You will see `forest` and then an `x` which the manual explains is *An object of class meta or metabind* which is a long way of saying the name of your meta-analysis, which you will recall is `MetaA`. The other arguments tell meta to add in tests of statistical significance for the fixed and random-effects model, respectively. You can have one, both or neither as you like, and to include them you type the argument followed by `TRUE`, like this `test.overall.fixed=TRUE, test.overall.random=TRUE`

So your code might look like this:

```
forest(MetaA, test.overall.fixed=TRUE, test.overall.
random=TRUE)
```

If you type this, then highlight it and press `control` and `R` together. It will open another window that contains your forest plot. You may have to resize it to see the whole plot.

This is not the prettiest, so we can do various things to make it look nicer:

```
forest(MetaA, test.overall.fixed=TRUE, test.over-
all.random=TRUE, digits =1, digits.sd=1, label.
left="Favours decaff", label.right="Favours caffiene")
```

This gives you a very pleasing forest plot as shown in Fig. B.1.

You will note that by default meta undertakes both fixed and random-effects models. There are good reasons for doing both as they mean slightly different things, but you can turn one or the other off if you like.

You can produce other plots such as:

```
funnel(MetaA)
radial(MetaA)
baujat(MetaA)
```

I won't spoil your surprise by doing them for you.

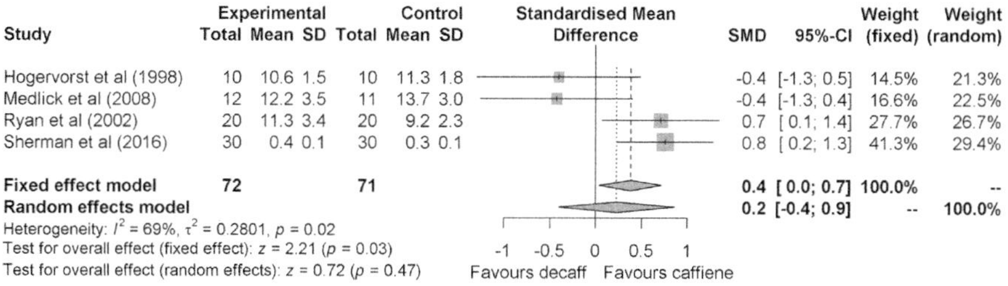

Study	Experimental Total Mean SD	Control Total Mean SD	Standardised Mean Difference	SMD	95%-CI	Weight (fixed)	Weight (random)
Hogervorst et al (1998)	10 10.6 1.5	10 11.3 1.8		-0.4	[-1.3; 0.5]	14.5%	21.3%
Medlick et al (2008)	12 12.2 3.5	11 13.7 3.0		-0.4	[-1.3; 0.4]	16.6%	22.5%
Ryan et al (2002)	20 11.3 3.4	20 9.2 2.3		0.7	[0.1; 1.4]	27.7%	26.7%
Sherman et al (2016)	30 0.4 0.1	30 0.3 0.1		0.8	[0.2; 1.3]	41.3%	29.4%
Fixed effect model	**72**	**71**		0.4	[0.0; 0.7]	100.0%	--
Random effects model				0.2	[-0.4; 0.9]	--	100.0%

Heterogeneity: $I^2 = 69\%$, $\tau^2 = 0.2801$, $p = 0.02$
Test for overall effect (fixed effect): $z = 2.21$ ($p = 0.03$)
Test for overall effect (random effects): $z = 0.72$ ($p = 0.47$)

-1   -0.5   0   0.5   1
Favours decaff   Favours caffiene

Fig. B.1 Forest plot

Multiple Effect Size Alert!

If you look back at the original data, you will see a potential problem with one study by Ryan which had two effect sizes.

Ryan et al. (2002)
Long-delay free recall (Morning)
caffeine mean = 11.8 (2.9), $n = 20$; decaffeinated mean = 11 (2.7), $n = 20$
Long-delay free recall (Afternoon)
caffeine mean = 11.7 (2.8), $n = 20$; decaffeinated mean = 8.9 (3), $n = 20$
A 20-min delay occurs next, followed by both free recall of the original list (long-delay free recall)

I took a very pragmatic option and chose one, but what if I wanted to use them both? What you can't do is include them both or simply average them. If you include them both as if they were separate studies that would lead to this study being over-weighted, both solutions make the assumption that the two entries are independent of each other which of course they are not; they are the same people tested twice. In this case, it did not matter to the direction of the effect (caffeine was better in both), but it did to the size of the difference between caffeine and decaffeinated coffee. There is a function in the MAd package called agg that will combine effect sizes; the problem is that you need to know the correlation between the effect sizes, and this is hardly ever reported.

This is a very brief introduction to meta-analysis using R and the meta package. There are lots of other things that you can do to examine your data further and beautify your plots. There are many other packages in R including:

metafor	This is a general package with a great deal of functionality; meta actually uses it. I used meta here rather than metafor because it produces plots more easily.
compute. es	This is a package that computes a variety of effect sizes including the standardised effect sizes d and g from a variety of other statistics.
bayesmeta	This undertakes Bayesian meta-analysis. If that does not mean anything to you, then you don't need to worry about it; you *would* know if you did!
MAd	This is a package that conducts meta-analysis on mean differences, it also contains the agg function for aggregating correlated effect sizes.

Graphics

To save the various plots, you can just right click and save them; R Studio has an **Export** button which allows you to export your graphic. The problem with these methods is that they will not give you a high-resolution plot, for publication you need to use graphic format-specific functions. This is a little beyond what we can cover in this chapter, but more information can be found on the internet. You can save your graphics in different formats including bmp, jpeg, pdf, ps and wmf.

This is the code used to produce the forest plot here:

```
tiff(file="forest.tiff", height=200, width=750)
forest(MetaB, test.overall.fixed=TRUE, test.overall.
random=TRUE, digits=1, digits.sd=1, label.left="Favours
decaff", label.right="Favours caffiene")
dev.off()
```

The tiff part says to produce a tiff file, the file= gives it a name (it will be saved on your hard disk using this name) and the height= and width= arguments say how big the plot should be. Try adjusting these to see what effect this has on the plot. This sometimes takes a little playing around with to get it right. You then run the forest function as before. Finally, the dev.off() argument turns the plotting device off.

Referencing R Packages

If you type `citation()` into R, it will tell you how to cite R, and if you type `citation("meta")` it will tell you how to cite the package (if you are using another package, simply change meta to the correct name).

R and R Packages

```
citation()
```

R Core Team (2019) R: a language and environment for statistical computing. R Foundation for Statistical Computing, Vienna. https://www.R-project.org/

```
citation("meta")
```

Schwarzer G (2007) meta: an R package for meta-analysis. R News 7(3):40–45

```
citation("metafor")
```

Viechtbauer W (2010) Conducting meta-analyses in R with the metafor package. J Stat Software 36(3):1–48. http://www.jstatsoft.org/v36/i03/

Other References

Hogervorst E, Riedel WJ, Schmitt JAJ, Jolles J (1998) Caffeine improves memory performance during distraction in middle-aged, but not in young or old subjects. Hum Psychopharmacol Clin Exp 13(4):277–284. https://doi.org/10.1002/(SICI)1099-1077(199806)13:4<277::AID-HUP996>3.0.CO;2-W

Mednick SC, Cai DJ, Kanady J, Drummond SPA (2008) Comparing the benefits of caffeine, naps and placebo on verbal, motor and perceptual memory. Behav Brain Res 193(1):79–86. https://doi.org/10.1016/j.bbr.2008.04.028

Ryan L, Hatfield C, Hofstetter M (2002) Caffeine reduces time-of-day effects on memory performance in older adults. Psychol Sci 13(1):68–71. https://doi.org/10.1111/1467-9280.00412

Sherman SM, Buckley TP, Baena E, Ryan L (2016) Caffeine enhances memory performance in young adults during their non-optimal time of day. Front Psychol 7

Now let us try and recreate the forest plot from Chap. 6. First here is the data, where Ab is those who took antibiotics and had a sore throat, Abn is the number in the antibiotic group, Pl the number in the placebo group with a sore throat and Pln the number in the placebo group.

Study	Ab	Abn	Pl	Pln
Brink (1951)	119	277	129	198
Brumfit (1957)	21	42	26	40
Chapple (1958)	40	135	37	65
Dagnelle (1996)	36	117	57	117
De Meyers (1992)	18	82	59	91
Denny (1953)	89	157	48	50
El Daher (1991)	42	111	106	118
Landsman (1951)	6	52	7	43
Little (1997)	135	215	122	187
MacDonald (1951)	18	41	27	41
Middleton (1966)	2	34	5	23
Petersen (1997)	60	89	74	90
Whitfield (1961)	129	258	165	272
Zwarl (2000)	215	358	131	164
Zwarl (2003)	79	100	38	56

Now run the code as before, but this time use the code for dichotomous data rather than continuous.

```
library(grid)
# You may need to download this package, it is not im-
portant but it adds the
# title
library(meta)
file.choose()
# Rember to find the .csv file location and to copy it in
below between the speech marks " "
dat<-read.csv(" ", header=TRUE)
MA1<-metabin(event.e=Ab, n.e=Abn, event.c=Pl, n.c=Pln,
data=dat, sm="RR", studlab=Study, label.left="Favours
antibiotics", label.right="Favours placebo")
# This undertakes the meta-anlaysis, remember before we
used metacont for
# continuous data?  Here we use metabin for binary or
dichotomous data
```

```
forest(MA1, test.overall.random  = TRUE, lab.
e="Antibiotics", lab.c="Placebo")
# This produces the forest plot as before
grid.text("Antibiotics v placebo - sore throat on day
3", .5, .93, gp=gpar(cex=1.5))
# This adds a title; if you find it a little high on the
page, reduce the .93 to .8 or however you prefer it
funnel(MA1)
# Funnel plot
funnel(MA1, contour = c(0.9, 0.95, 0.99),
studlab=dat$Study, col.contour=c("dark grey", "grey",
"light grey"), pos.studlab=4) legend("topright",
legend=c("0.1 > p > 0.05", "0.05 > p > 0.01", "< 0.01"),
fill=c("dark grey", "grey", "light grey"), bg="white",
ce=0.8)
# This produces the funnel plot with the 'contours'
showing levels of
# statistical significance
metabias(MA1)
trim<-trimfill(MA1, studlab=TRUE)
funnel(trim)
# The trim and fill analysis and plot
forest(MA1, layout = "RevMan5")
# Now make it look like the output from RevMan - the
Cochrane software
```

Reference

Brink WRR, Denny FW, Wannamaker LW (1951) Effect of penicillin and aureomycin on the natural course of streptococcal tonsillitis and pharyngitis. Am J Med
10:300–308.

Appendix C: Using GRADEpro Guideline Development Tool

Using GRADEpro GDT

GRADEpro GDT (GDT stands for Guideline Development Tool) is a web-based application for use by authors of healthcare guidelines which you can find here https://gradepro.org/ (GRADEpro GDT 2015). Although it has a high degree of integration with the Cochrane software RevMan, it can be used as we will do so here with other software. The licence allows free and unrestricted use of any non-commercial projects. Although either on its own, or in combination with RevMan, it allows for the development of guidance from review right through to recommendation; here we will use it just for producing a GRADE **Evidence Profile** and a **Summary of Findings** table. We begin by entering GRADEpro. If you have used RevMan, your questions can be directly imported into the programme, if not we need to enter it by hand. This is no more complicated than selecting the Comparisons tab on the left-hand side and then choosing the type of question that you have and then entering the question. When you add an outcome, different parts of the table will be activated depending on your choice of data type. These can be either continuous, dichotomous, time to event or narrative; and whether the data are pooled, not pooled, a range of effects, a single study, not measured, or not reported. When you add in results, many of the calculations within the table are done for you, and those which are not relevant are not active.

For example, in our meta-analysis, we have continuous data that have been pooled. We begin by entering the standardised mean difference and its confidence interval into the box headed **Anticipated absolute effects (95% CI)**. Because we have included studies using different scales in our meta-analysis (this is why we are using the standardised rather than raw mean difference), we can't enter the mean score in the control group **Without Caffeine** box which is generally useful to help us understand the magnitude of effect and importance of the outcome. What we can put in however is the standardised mean difference and its confidence interval which shows the absolute change in the score. After that we can then calculate the **Certainty** of the effect using the GRADE criteria which we discussed in Chap. 9, but this time it will be a more sophisticated calculation because it contains a number of different levels for each criteria.

The levels are:

© The Editor(s) (if applicable) and The Author(s), under exclusive license to Springer Nature Switzerland AG 2020
E. Purssell, N. McCrae, *How to Perform a Systematic Literature Review*, https://doi.org/10.1007/978-3-030-49672-2

Risk of bias: Not serious, Serious, Very Serious
Inconsistency: Not serious, Serious, Very Serious
Indirectness: Not serious, Serious, Very Serious
Imprecision: Not serious, Serious, Very Serious
Publication bias: Undetected, Strongly Suspected
Large effect: No, Large, Very Large
Plausible confounding: No, Would Reduce Demonstrated Effect, Would Suggest Spurious Effect
Dose response effect: No, Yes.

Having entered these in the **Certainty** column, the score will be calculated and displayed. In our case that has come out as Very Low. You also have the option (which you should take up) to add **footnotes** explaining your decisions. You can then use one of the generated **What happens** statements, or write one of your own.

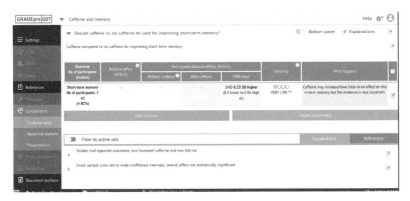

Then you can also export the completed **Evidence Profile**

and the **Summary of Findings table**

Appendix D: Interpreting Effect Sizes

Often in this book we have referred to the size of the effect. Sometimes this is clear, but where outcomes are not in natural units of measurement, such as the standardised effect size, which is not always easily interpretable this guidance may be useful (Table D.1).

Table D.1 Guidance for configuration of qualitative and quantitative findings

Value	Standardised effect size (e.g. Cohen's d) (Cohen 1988)	Sawilowsky (2009)—new effect size rules of thumb (e.g. d)	Correlation r (Cohen 1988)	Ferguson (2009)—ES primer or RR	Description
0	0		0		No relationship or difference
0.5		0.01		2[a]	Very small positive result
1	0.2	0.2	0.1		Small or weak positive result
2	0.5	0.5	0.3	3	Medium or moderate positive result
3	0.8	0.8	0.5	4	Large or strong positive result
4		1.2			Very large positive result
5		2			Huge positive result

[a]Minimum effect size representing a practically significant effect of social science data

References

Cohen J (1988) Statistical power analysis for the behavioral sciences, 2nd edn. L. Erlbaum Associates, Hillsdale, NJ

Ferguson CJ (2009) An effect size primer: a guide for clinicians and researchers. Prof Psychol Res Pract 40:532–538. https://doi.org/10.1037/a0015808

GRADEpro GDT (2015) GRADEpro Guideline Development Tool [Software]. https://gradepro.org/. Accessed 6 Mar 2020

Sawilowsky SS (2009) New effect size rules of thumb. J Mod App Stat Meth 8:597–599. https://doi.org/10.22237/jmasm/1257035100

© The Editor(s) (if applicable) and The Author(s), under exclusive license to Springer Nature Switzerland AG 2020
E. Purssell, N. McCrae, *How to Perform a Systematic Literature Review*,
https://doi.org/10.1007/978-3-030-49672-2

Glossary

Analysis Thorough examination of a set of data or findings.

Association A generally perceived relationship between variables, not necessarily supported by evidence.

Bayesian statistics A branch of statistical inference that uses prior knowledge alongside data to calculate the full posterior distribution of the parameter of interest. It is not covered in this book. Most statistics make use of frequentist methods.

Bias A systematic error, likely to detract from the truth.

Bibliographic database An organised collection of published literature, often specialised (e.g. medicine). These include Medline/PubMed, Embase and PsycInfo.

Boolean operator A word used to connect or exclude search terms (e.g. and, or, not).

Case–control study A study that recruits a group of participants with a particular condition, alongside a group of participants without the condition. Cases and controls are then compared on the outcome of interest. Such a design is often used for rare illnesses or events.

Case report An account of a single patient.

Case series An account of a set of patients with a similarity (typically having the same illness or treatment). Like a single case report, the information is descriptive rather than the product of scientific study.

CASP Critical Appraisal Skills Programme. A source of critical appraisal tools.

Causation An observed causal relationship between variables (cause and effect).

CERQual Confidence in the Evidence from Reviews of Qualitative research is a tool for assessing the confidence that can be placed in the findings from a qualitative systematic review. It is associated with GRADE.

Clinical significance A judgement on whether study findings are clinically important. Note that a result can be statistically significant but not clinically significant (and *vice versa*).

Cochrane Previously known as the Cochrane Collaboration, this is an international and independent network of researchers, methodologists and practitioners with the mission of enhancing evidence-based healthcare.

© The Editor(s) (if applicable) and The Author(s), under exclusive license to Springer Nature Switzerland AG 2020
E. Purssell, N. McCrae, *How to Perform a Systematic Literature Review*,
https://doi.org/10.1007/978-3-030-49672-2

Cohort study A study that follows a group of people over a period of time. Cohort studies can be prospective or retrospective, but either way, participants are not recruited on the basis of an outcome.

Comparator A group used for comparison against a group having the intervention/exposure of interest. Having a broader definition than a control group, a comparator group may receive a different treatment, or the same treatment as the intervention group but of different dose or duration. There may be multiple comparators in a study.

Conclusion An overarching statement of the findings and implications of a study/review.

Confidence interval An estimate, computed from observed data, of a range of plausible values for a parameter.

CONSORT Consolidated Standards of Reporting Trials. A reporting guideline for randomised controlled trials.

ConQual A tool for establishing confidence in the output of qualitative research synthesis. Particularly associated with the Joanna Briggs Institute.

Control group A group of participants who are as similar as possible to the experimental group, differing only on the intervention/exposure of interest. By experimental convention this group receives a placebo, but if this is not feasible, a control group in a quasi-experimental design may receive no treatment (or usual care).

Correlation An observed relationship between variables. Take care not to confuse correlation with causation.

Credibility Used in qualitative research to assess the 'fit' between the original data and the author's interpretation. Sometimes seen to be analogous with internal validity.

Credible interval Most often found in Bayesian statistics, which are not covered in this book. This is what most people incorrectly think a confidence interval is. This is an interval within which the population parameter value falls with a given probability. For example, it might be the range within which you can be 95% confident a particular population value lies.

Critical appraisal In systematic reviewing, this means evaluating the quality of studies, normally using a critical appraisal tool.

Cross-sectional study An observational study that analyses data from a population at a single time point.

Dependability Used in qualitative research to assess the extent to which the research or review process is logical, trackable, and is clearly documented and able to be followed. Sometimes seen to be analogous with reliability.

Diagnosis A judgement of the medical condition that explains or may explain the patient's symptoms.

Discussion Examination by argument.

Effect size The result of what was measured in a study, in the unit of measurement applied (e.g. mmHg for blood pressure). Not to be confused with standardised effect size.

Effectiveness Whether an intervention works under normal clinical circumstances. This may be investigated by observational studies.

Efficacy Whether an intervention works under ideal or experimental circumstances, as in a randomised controlled trial.

Eligibility criteria Determinants of which people, time period or conditions qualify for a study/review.

Empirical From observation rather than theory. Qualitative and quantitative methods are empirical forms of enquiry.

Epidemiology A branch of medicine concerned with incidence, distribution and causes of illness.

EQUATOR network Enhancing the Quality and Transparency of Health Research. A website with various guidelines for reporting research.

Ethnography A qualitative research method whereby researchers observe or engage in a cultural group, exploring customs and beliefs from group members' perspectives.

Evidence The available facts or information indicating the validity of a contribution to knowledge.

Exclusion criteria Disqualifications for a study/review (e.g. participants too young, or studies without control groups)

Experimental study A scientific investigation conducted in controlled conditions.

Exposure An experience or opportunity/risk of an experience investigated in research, normally over a specified time period.

Facet analysis The dividing of elements from a field of knowledge into constituent parts, and sorting into a meaningful structure with appropriate labels.

Fixed-effects model In a meta-analysis, a model assuming that all studies are measuring the same true effect and that any difference in outcome is due to variation in samples (therefore, if all studies had sufficiently large samples, the results would be similar).

Forest plot A graphical representation used in meta-analysis, showing the result of each study with pooled estimate and confidence interval.

Frequentist statistics A branch of statistics where probabilities are based on the long-term frequency of getting a particular result. For example, a probability of 0.05 means that one would expect to get this result in 5% of trials if the study were to be repeated many times.

Funnel plot A scatterplot of treatment effect against a measure of study precision.

GRADE Grading of Recommendations for Assessment, Development and Evaluation. This is a method for transparently grading the quality of evidence and giving a strength to recommendations based on it.

Grey literature Reports not published in peer-reviewed journals and thus not indexed in scientific databases. Examples are policy documents, survey reports by voluntary organisations and scientific research not submitted to journals (for whatever reason).

Grounded theory An optimally inductive method of qualitative research, generating theory from the data.

Heterogeneity In the context of a review, this means variation between the studies (methodological, clinical or statistical). In meta-analysis, it means whether studies are measuring the same (homogeneity) or different (heterogeneity) effect underlying true effect.

Hierarchy of evidence An ordering of knowledge that prioritises experimental over observational studies, quantitative over qualitative and scientific investigation over expert opinion or anecdote. The value of such hierarchies is contested.

Homogeneity In reviewing research, this means studies being similar (in methods, participants or results). For meta-analysis, see heterogeneity (above).

Hypothesis A speculated relationship between variables of interest, to be tested by scientific investigation, typically comparing a treated/exposed group with a control group.

I^2 Percentage of variation across studies in a meta-analysis that is thought to be due to heterogeneity rather than chance.

Implication A conclusion that can reasonably be drawn from a study/review.

Incidence The number of instances of a condition occurring in a specified period of time.

Inclusion criteria Qualifications for a study/review (e.g. age of participants, types of study).

Interpretative In qualitative research, exploring the meaning of a perspective or experience to study participants, individually and possibly collectively (depending on the method).

Intervention A treatment or other activity under investigation.

Linear Following a sequential process from one stage to next.

Literature In the context of a systematic review, any document that reports or reviews research. Normally, it is required that such literature appears in a peer-reviewed journal.

Logic Reasoning by robust argument, expressed in valid or proven statements.

MeSH Medical Subject Headings (as used in PubMed database). This is a set of headings under which papers are indexed.

Meta-analysis Statistical aggregation of studies for analysis.

Meta-regression An extension of the statistical method of regression to investigate whether a moderating variable has an effect on study results in a meta-analysis.

Metasynthesis A method for reviewing qualitative research findings.

Method The process of a study/review.

Methodology A theoretical discussion of methods, often to present a rationale for a study design.

Mixed method Research entailing more than one method; typically meaning a combination of qualitative and quantitative methods. A mixed-method review may include qualitative, quantitative and mixed-method studies.

Narrative review A loosely-used term for a review of studies and their findings, which does not entail statistical analysis. A systematic narrative review is a rigorous and explicit examination of studies.

Negative May mean something that is not beneficial, or a relationship between variables that is refuted by evidence. This is a problematic term because it is sometimes used to mean no difference (e.g. a drug is equivalent to placebo in outcome), and sometimes an undesirable difference (e.g. a drug produces a worse outcome).

Null hypothesis The hypothesis that there is no difference in outcome between a treated/exposed group and a control group.

Outcome Result of a studied intervention/exposure.

P **value** The probability of getting a study result (or a result more extreme) if the null-hypothesis is true. It is not the probability that the result has occurred by chance, whatever some research manuals suggest!

Parameter A number that describes a population (e.g. mean, variance).

Peer review The convention in academic journals whereby submitted study reports are evaluated by researchers/scholars in the same field as the author.

Phenomenon Something that is perceived/experienced.

Phenomenology A qualitative research method that explores individual human experience in depth.

PICO Population, intervention, control and outcome. A configuration for demarcating the scope, eligibility criteria and search terms for a review.

Placebo In an experimental trial, a dummy treatment that appears the same as the treatment, so that participants, practitioners and researchers can be blinded to allocation.

Placebo effect Improvement perceived by a trial participant despite receiving an inert substance (placebo), due to belief in the treatment.

Point estimate A single number that summarises the result of a study, using the primary outcome measurement (e.g. mean mmHg).

Pooled estimate Result of a meta-analysis, from the pooled results of studies, estimating a parameter in the wider population.

Population The group of people from whom a sample is really or theoretically drawn, and to whom a study result is generalised.

Positive May mean something that is beneficial, or a relationship between variables verified by evidence (often both apply; e.g. a tested treatment that relieves symptoms).

Prevalence The number of people with a particular condition at a specified time point.

Primary outcome measurement The most important indicator of the effect of the studied intervention/exposure, always determined at the outset.

PRISMA Preferred Reporting Items for Systematic Reviews and Meta-Analyses. The reporting guidelines that most peer-reviewed journals expect reviewers to follow.

Prognosis The likely course of a medical condition.

Q **statistic** In meta-analysis, the weighted sum of squared differences between individual study effects and the pooled effect across studies. The associated p-value is a test of heterogeneity, with a p-value of <0.1 often used as grounds to reject the null hypothesis of homogeneity and so indicative of heterogeneity.

Qualitative In research, investigating the meaning of experience (phenomena).

Quality A word with various meanings. In reviewing research, it is an evaluation of the rigour and credibility of study findings.

Quantitative Measuring something by number.

Quasi-experiment An intervention study lacking randomisation but otherwise adhering to experimental design.

Random allocation Participants are randomly allocated to treatment/exposure or control groups, so that any differences between groups are due to chance.

Random-effects model In meta-analysis, this model does not assume that all studies are measuring the same true effect, but instead takes the studies as a sample from a larger 'population' of studies, all with slightly different true effects. Variation in these true effects are measured by heterogeneity statistics.

Randomised controlled trial This is the classic experimental design, having three defining features: randomisation, manipulation of a variable and a control group. Blinding is used to mask random assignment, thereby minimising bias.

Reference management tool Applications such as EndNote enable researchers to create and manage records of relevant literature. In reviewing, these tools are useful for managing search results and for screening.

Regression A type of statistical analysis used to measure relationships between one or more independent variables and a dependent variable.

Reliability The extent to which a study produces a result that would be consistent with other studies conducted in similar conditions.

Reporting guidelines Tools to guide researchers, editors and reviewers on the essential information to be presented in a study report. These are design-specific (e.g. CONSORT for randomised controlled trials).

Review question The aim of a review, stated as a specific question to be answered by examining relevant studies.

Rigour Quality and trustworthiness of a study/review, which should be conducted systematically.

Risk of bias tool An instrument to assess the risk of bias in a study, or in a review.

ROBIS Risk of Bias in Systematic Reviews. A widely used tool for assessing bias in a systematic review.

Sample The group of participants in a study.

Sampling The process of recruiting a sample. In a probability sample, everyone in the population has a known and equal chance of being in the sample; hence, it is random. Most samples in healthcare research are not really probability samples. Probably, the most common type of sampling is convenience sampling, which is simply recruiting people who happen to be there. However, most statistical tests assume a random sample!

Sampling error Variation arising from sampling. Each random sample from the same population will produce different results because each set of people is different. This variation is known as sampling error. Generally, the larger the sample the smaller the sampling error. Many statistical tests are based on estimating how much of an effect is real and how much is due to sampling error.

Screening The process of checking the eligibility of studies found by the search.

Searching The process of searching the literature, mostly by automated application of search terms, but also can include manual methods such as trawling reference lists of papers.

SPIDER Sample, phenomenon of interest, design, evaluation, research type. A configuration for demarcating the scope, eligibility criteria and search terms for a review of qualitative research.

Standard deviation A measure of the distribution of data points in a sample. It is of most use if the data are normally distributed; if so, 95% of the data points will be within a range of plus or minus 1.96 standard deviations from the mean value. The mean plus and minus 1.96 standard deviations gives a 95% confidence interval for the sample.

Standard error A measure of how accurately a statistic based on a sample estimates the population parameter. If the same study were repeated infinitely, and each time a 95% confidence interval was calculated, 95% of these intervals would include the true value. The confidence threshold may be set at 99% or at a lower level. Not to be confused with the standard deviation or the credible interval.

Standardised effect size An effect size with unit of measurement removed, allowing different measurements from studies to be combined.

Statistical power A measure of the likelihood of a study to reject the null hypothesis (should this be false).

Statistical significance This is often linked to the p value. If p is below a specified threshold (typically 0.05), the data are considered incompatible with the null hypothesis, and the null hypothesis is therefore rejected.

STROBE Strengthening the Reporting of Observational Studies in Epidemiology. A reporting guideline for most types of observational study.

Summary statistic A number that summarises a set of data or results (e.g. mean score on a pain assessment scale). To make sense of the summary statistic, a measure of variation or precision is also needed.

Synthesis Combination of analysed data or findings to produce an overall conclusion.

Systematic Following a set of procedures rigorously.

Theme A concept interpreted from qualitative data.

Type I error Rejecting the null hypothesis when it is true, producing a 'false positive'. This may be attributable to an excessive sample size.

Type II error Failing to reject a false null hypothesis, producing a 'false negative'. This may be attributable to an insufficient sample size.

Validity Comprised of two aspects. Internal validity is the extent to which a result is likely to be free of bias. External validity refers to the ability to apply the results scientific beyond the context of the specific study.

Variable Something with a quality or quantity that varies.

Vote counting A method of combining studies by simply counting the number of studies with each outcome. It is normally not recommended because it does not entail weighting of studies, and it does not provide a pooled estimate, confidence interval or heterogeneity statistics.

Weighting In meta-analysis, a method of allowing some studies to contribute more to the pooled estimate than others. In a fixed-effects model, the weighting is based on the inverse of variance; in the random-effects model, it is based on the inverse of variance and an estimate of heterogeneity. This makes the fixed-effects model more susceptible to differences in sample size, while in the random-effects model the studies are more balanced.

Subject Index

Author Index

© The Editor(s) (if applicable) and The Author(s), under exclusive license to Springer
Nature Switzerland AG 2020
E. Purssell, N. McCrae, *How to Perform a Systematic Literature Review*,
https://doi.org/10.1007/978-3-030-49672-2

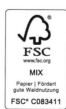